The Medical School Manual

Also by Sujay Kansagra, MD:

Everything I Learned in Medical School: Besides All the Book Stuff

Why Medicine? And 500 Other Questions for the Medical School and Residency Interviews

My Child Won't Sleep: A Quick Guide for the Sleep-Deprived Parent

THE MEDICAL SCHOOL MANUAL
Getting in, Staying in, and Thriving

Sujay M. Kansagra, MD

ISBN-13: 9781072083863

To everyone who will go on this journey.

Contents

Preface

In 2011, a wave of uprisings spread through the Arab world. Civilians clashed with their governments. Protestors demanded change. Entire regimes were overthrown. It was an unprecedented, united front among a massive group of people seeking relief from oppressive governments. The media in the United States pointed to a variety of contributing factors that led to the uprisings. Yet one factor stood out as a prominent force among these protesters—the use of social media.

Protestors were organizing as never before thanks to the common link of social media. Twitter in particular would often receive credit and was quickly becoming a worldwide phenomenon. It invaded everyday life. You couldn't get far in your day without seeing references to a hashtag. Not wanting to be left behind in the new trend, I joined. My goal was to contribute to this microblogging, worldwide forum in a positive way. Because my expertise was in medical school education, I decided I would share advice for current and future students. My Twitter handle became @Medschooladvice.

"Maybe I'll get a few hundred followers if I'm lucky," I thought to myself.

Seven years and more than 120,000 followers later, my account has become the most popular source for medical school advice on Twitter. Students and professionals from around the world have tuned in for the discussion. I've learned as much from my followers as they have learned from me.

Unfortunately Twitter was often a bit constraining for sharing advice. The reason is simple: great advice often takes more than 280 characters. I knew I had much more I could share to help premedical and medical students on their journey, and thus this book was born.

If there is one piece of advice I can impart before we even get started, it's to realize how different we all are and how rarely one piece of advice will apply to everyone equally. The points highlighted in this book represent an approach that worked for me and one that I feel would be beneficial for the majority of students. However, life has no guarantees, and admission to medical school is no exception.

The journey to becoming a doctor can feel confusing, overwhelming, and frightening. My hope is that this book will offer you guidance on your journey. But no one can determine your course. You alone will decide where the path takes you. I wish you nothing but the best on your journey.

Section I
High School

This section is dedicated to high school students interested in becoming physicians. The goal is to provide avenues through which you may explore the field and to set you on the path to success when applying to college.

Chapter 1

When Grades Start to Matter

Believe it or not, up until the start of high school, your grades have not mattered. That's not to say grades were not important in elementary and middle school. On the contrary, your performance in school thus far likely reflects how you will end up doing in high school and beyond. However, when it comes to your future prospects of gaining admission into college and subsequently into medical school, your elementary and middle school performance will not play a role simply because it is not a part of your college applications. So consider high school a blank slate. If you have not done well in the past, now is the time to get your act together. If you have been a straight-A student, work to continue this trend.

Because your college applications will highlight both your class rank and GPA, this is the time to put your best foot forward. A strong academic performance will be vital toward obtaining admission and scholarships.

Not only are grades important in high school, so are the types of courses you take. Those who intend to go on the premed track in college should be taking challenging and rigorous courses in high school. Particularly, taking multiple Advanced Placement (AP)/International Baccalaureate (IB) courses will not only boost class rank should you get an A, but these courses may also provide useful credits you can apply toward college if you pass the AP/IB exam at the end of the year. Having such credits in college can make your schedule much more flexible.

How many advanced courses should you take? Every high school is different and offers a varying number of advanced courses. First, determine how many you feel comfortable taking based on the workload. Then, try to develop a sense of how many advanced courses may be necessary to rank well in your graduating class. This strategy will obviously depend on what everybody else is taking and how your school determines class rank. For my high school, taking eight AP courses and making straight A's put students in the top five of my graduating class of 400 students. However, competition has become more rigorous since I graduated; it is not unusual for students to start taking AP courses as early as freshman year of high school. But more important than the number of advanced courses is your performance. There is no point to taking many advanced courses if you don't get good grades in them.

Given the rigors of high school, this is also a great time to find healthy competition. Being competitive often brings out the absolute best in individuals. History is filled with examples of how competition has led to greatness: Picasso versus Matisse, Steve Jobs versus Bill Gates, and Michelangelo versus Leonardo da Vinci. Having someone to compete against adds to your drive and determination. You certainly do not have to be unfriendly and turn high school into a contest. However, finding a group of students who are as equally motivated as you often helps drive all of you to achieve your goals. Some of my best friends in high school were also the ones I competed against the most. We brought each other up rather than tried to bring one another down. Competition and friendship do not need to be mutually exclusive.

So take a deep breath as you begin high school, find some healthy competition, and prepare to work hard. This is when it really starts to count. Let's explore ways to make you a high school star in the next few chapters.

Chapter 2

Study Tips

What does it take to finish among the top few in your graduating class? Some students are naturally brilliant and never have to put much effort into studying. But for most of us, getting good grades entails persistence and a diligent work ethic. And just as important is an effective and efficient approach to studying.

The majority of learning in high school is rote memorization. Good test takers are the ones who can memorize thoroughly and simply recall this information at test time. If you dedicate enough time to memorizing the materials, chances are you will do well. Except for a select few classes, not much room exists for abstract thinking and critical evaluation during high school. This situation is particularly true in the science courses. That's good news for the particularly obsessive students who ensure they memorize everything perfectly prior to examinations. The fact is that you do need to be a little obsessive to succeed in high school, college, and the field of medicine. So do not fight this tendency to obsess; embrace it. It will serve you well. Of course, don't overly obsess. Try your best to enjoy high school and spend time doing activities other than studying. In fact a well-rounded person makes a much more attractive candidate to potential colleges. See chapter 4 on extracurriculars for more on this perspective.

What are the other factors to doing well in high school classes? Here are a few of my tips:

1. Plan ahead. Don't spend the night before each test staying up until four o'clock in the morning. Instead start studying a few days earlier to give yourself time to digest the material fully. Granted, you likely may have a few classes where you can get away with cramming just the night before, but for many, the material will be too extensive. Similarly commit yourself to studying as soon as you come home from school each day. Complete your assignments and studying as early as possible. If you wait until the evening, you may find that you've misjudged the amount of work and end up sacrificing sleep.

2. Avoid distractions. This is probably the most important piece of advice and likely the hardest one to follow. High school students these days have a thousand different distractions trying to fight for a small piece of attention. E-mail, Snapchat, Instagram, Twitter, texting...distractions are everywhere. And unfortunately they all follow you wherever you go

thanks to the smartphone. And although keeping up with texts and posting your latest selfies on Instagram may seem incredibly important, in the long run you will likely look back and regret the time you wasted. Fight the temptation to let social media and other distractions take over your world.

3. Use memory tricks. We all know how useful mnemonics can be when learning. Take things a step further and use your visual memory. See chapter 25, where I teach you the best memory trick ever! For those who still prefer the rote memorization approach, flash cards are a great way to commit new information to memory. Be sure to put small bits of information on each card. Set cards aside once you have learned them, and only go through cards yet to be learned. Once you are through all of the cards, mix them up and repeat the process.

4. Avoid too much time in study groups. Studying in a group is usually inefficient. You end up talking more about the latest gossip than the study material. And if you happen to be the smartest person in the group, you will likely not learn anything new during these sessions. Study alone for the majority of the time. Studying with a group is reasonable for the extra motivation it provides. Teaching others is also a great

way to cement your own knowledge. But these groups should not be your principal studying method.

5. Keep questioning yourself. After you read over the material, ask yourself what you have learned. Try to think about how you would explain it to others. Don't get into the habit of superficial studying, in which you simply read and highlight the material but don't actively think about it.

I encourage you to read over the section on study strategies in chapter 23 for more tips on how to become an efficient studying machine.

In addition to studying efficiently, here are some other keys to coming out on top when high school is over.

1. Stay organized. Use a calendar to keep track of assignments and upcoming tests. Too much happens in high school to remember everything. Staying organized makes it much more manageable and prevents you from feeling overwhelmed.

2. Make a good impression. Don't be a class clown with hopes of winning your classmates' affection. Your teachers really can make your time in school difficult if they choose. On the other hand, teachers can also be your biggest source of support. So make a good

impression from the start. Show them that you are hardworking and take classes seriously no matter the subject. You'll be surprised how much a teacher's attitude toward you will influence your final grade no matter how objective teachers think they may be. And remember you will need recommendations when you apply for college and scholarships.

3. Get some sleep. High school students are notorious for staying up late and the next day struggling through the first few classes. Then on weekends they sleep until noon to make up for the sleep deprivation from the school week. This path to learning is very inefficient. Bad sleep hygiene that starts in high school will follow you throughout all of your future education. High school students typically need about nine hours of sleep every night! Studies show that the more students sleep, the better they perform in school. So try to get the nine hours you need. Avoid late-night exposure to bright lights from TVs, laptops, and smartphones, which can make sleeping harder. Try to keep your bedtime and wake time the same the entire week, including weekends. This can be tricky in high school, and everyone is entitled to stay up late to have a social life. But on days when you have the choice, choose sleep.

Hopefully these bits of advice will help you obtain a strong GPA, which is the cornerstone to a strong college application. Next we will talk about the second most important aspect of a strong application—your standardized test scores.

<u>Chapter 3</u>

Taking the SAT/ACT

If there is one thing you'll get to know well on your journey to becoming a doctor, it's the standardized test. This type of exam will continue for the remainder of your life if you have a career in medicine. But with the proper preparation, these tests can actually become quite rewarding and even fun (yes, fun).

The key to any standardized test is not just a thorough study of the material being tested, but also practice, practice, and more practice. The SAT and ACT are no different. Most colleges require one or the other to gain admission. Research your particular schools of interest to determine which test they require. Not sure which colleges you're interested in? Plan to take both tests. Different colleges use these test scores in different ways. Some weigh the results very highly, while others rely more on your academic performance in high school. Either way, thoroughly preparing for the examinations to obtain the best score possible is vital.

For either test I strongly recommend that you buy a review book that will guide you through the material and give you an overview of the exam format. You will find book suggestions at the end of the chapter. You should be intimately aware of how the exam is structured, including exactly which topics are covered, how many sections are in the exam, how many questions are in each section, and the time limits. Most review books will also have a section of practice questions. I recommend doing as many practice questions as humanly possible prior to taking a standardized test. Let me repeat—practice!

One of the biggest mistakes people make for the SAT and ACT is waiting too long before they take it. Some students take the test for the first time during their senior year. I highly advise against this. The great thing about both of these exams is that you can take them numerous times and yet only send your best score to your designated colleges. There are a few rare exceptions in which the college requests all scores, but they should use your highest scores to judge the application. So taking these tests multiple times is to your advantage. I took the pre-SAT (PSAT) for the first time in seventh grade and continued studying for the real thing until my senior year of college. I ended up taking the SAT four or five times. I blew the top off of the exam. Yet I took the ACT just once and studied only during my senior year. I scored mediocre. It is obvious that my performance had more to do with my preparation than my intelligence. Need more proof? The official ACT page reports that of the students who took the ACT more than once, 57 percent increased their score, 21 percent had no change, and 22 percent did worse. With only 22 percent of students doing worse, why wouldn't you take it again? Even if you do worse, simply send your first score.

Be sure to ask your school if it allows you to take the PSAT in the ninth and tenth grades for practice. It is typically offered in the eleventh grade, but you may be able to take it earlier. It is a shortened version of the SAT, but it will provide you with a score and a report of overall performance. This will give you a great sense of where you stand going into your junior and senior years.

Keep in mind that some institutions will require SAT subject tests in addition to the SAT. Check their websites early in your high school years so you can plan accordingly.

Many companies offer courses to help you prepare for the SAT and ACT. These courses may be helpful in terms of establishing structure to your learning, but they can also hurt your pocketbook. Look for free courses offered through your high school and buy a thorough study guide. Regardless of whether you take a course, a thorough study guide that covers core material is vital.

What study guide do I recommend? Times have changed quite a bit from when I took the SAT. The following suggestions are based on the recommendations from my Twitter followers. All book suggestions are ranked based on votes from Twitter. I also list some helpful websites and smartphone apps to help you prepare for the SAT and ACT.

SAT

Books:

1. *The Official SAT Study Guide* by The College Board
2. *Barron's SAT* by Sharon Weiner Green, MA, and Ira K. Wolf, PhD
3. *Barron's SAT 1600* by Linda Carnevale, MA, and Roselyn Teukolsky, MS

Websites:

http://sat.collegeboard.org: The official page for the SAT. Find more information about the test, test dates, and sample questions.

www.khanacademy.org/test-prep/sat: A great site for learning anything, SAT included. Here you will find a full-length test and video tutorials with explanations to many of the questions.

http://pwntestprep.com: Created by a guy who has destroyed every standardized test he has taken, this site shares tips and tricks on mastering the SAT.

Smartphone Apps:

Daily Practice for the SAT: This app gives you a question every day from each section of the SAT. It's a nice way for those smartphone lovers to get a little extra studying done during a free minute or two. The questions have to be good because they come straight from the writers of the SAT.

SAT Up: Loads of practice content with detailed explanations.

ACT

Books:

1. *The Real ACT* (Real ACT Prep Guide) by ACT Inc.
2. *Cracking the ACT* by Princeton Review
3. *Barron's ACT 36: Aiming for the Perfect Score* by Alexander Spare, MA, and Ann Hirsch, MA

Websites:

www.actstudent.org: The official page for the ACT. Has information on registering for the test, test dates, test preparation information, and more.

www.sparknotes.com/testprep: Provides an overview of the test with great strategies. Also has content for the SAT.

Smartphone Apps:

ACT Up: Offers many practice questions, personalized training, and games to help expand your vocabulary.

ACT Ace: Lots of digital flash cards to help familiarize yourself with the content of the exam.

Have more suggestions? Tweet me @medschooladvice.

Chapter 4

Choosing Extracurricular Activities

Having a competitive application to college isn't easy. Not only do you have to get good grades and perform well on standardized testing, you are also expected to participate in a variety of extracurricular activities throughout high school. Every college and scholarship application will ask you about these activities. Having both quantity and quality for this section is important. Quantity is important because applications will often have allotted space to list all of your activities, and being able to fill the available space is nice. Many will even allow you to attach additional sheets to the application to list all of your activities. However, quality is also important because you will likely encounter essay questions that ask about your most meaningful experiences. Having one or two main activities in which you are particularly active is vital. Here are the broad categories for extracurricular activities.

Volunteer Activities

Volunteering your time is important during high school. It shows good moral character and can be a very rewarding activity. Where you volunteer is not as important as simply volunteering. For those interested in medical school, I do recommend volunteering at a hospital for at least some period of time. Doing this can give you experience with patient interaction. However, volunteering in the hospital is not likely to provide much insight into a life in medicine because the assigned activities are vastly different than medical student or physician duties. However, you may be able to speak with doctors to get a better sense of their routines and paths to becoming physicians. Most large hospitals have volunteer programs already in place that you can simply contact to get the process going.

Many students confuse shadowing with volunteering. Volunteering is an activity in which you are helping others in some way. During shadowing you simply follow around a physician while that professional sees patients. Although this route can be a helpful experience for a student, I would not consider shadowing a substantial extracurricular activity. This is simply because you are not doing anything while shadowing. You are not helping others in any way. Shadowing is more beneficial to you than anyone else. So do not spend too much time shadowing. Regardless of how many hours you dedicate to shadowing, it will still only be one line on your applications. I would recommend just a few hours at this stage in your life, and ideally it should be a part of a formal premedical program that you can list as an extracurricular.

Organizations/Clubs

Not only will you be asked to list groups with which you are involved, you will also be asked to list leadership positions within these organizations. I would encourage you to run for positions in various clubs and student government. Having leadership positions shows that you made a substantial contribution and are not afraid to take charge. These are the types of people colleges want.

Sports

Participating in a sport is considered a great extracurricular activity. It shows that you can be a member of a team and know the importance of teamwork. If you have a sport you enjoy, try to join the high school or extramural team. You don't have to be a sports star. Participation alone is important.

Science Fairs and Other Academic Contests

Science Olympiad, Odyssey of the Mind, and math contests are just a few examples. Taking part in them is an easy way to grow your list of extracurriculars. Just participating is significant. Winning or getting an award is even better.

The most important thing to realize is that there are no "right" extracurricular activities. You should strive to participate in activities that you enjoy and can contribute to in a significant way.

My last piece of advice on extracurriculars is also the most important. Make a list! There is no way to remember all of your activities after four years of high school when it comes time to put together your application. Start a list as soon as possible—even in middle school—and add to the list every time you participate in something new. Do not wait a week or a month to update the list, update it just as soon as you participate in a new activity. Put everything on this list whether you feel it was important or not. Even spending one afternoon volunteering in the soup kitchen is worth noting. Write it all down!

How many activities should you participate in? This question has no right answer. If you want to be a serious applicant for top colleges and scholarships, the answer is a lot. Try to participate in as many worthwhile activities as possible. Having a list of at least ten different activities, leadership positions, sports, academic competitions, or honors/awards per year of high school is a good start.

Chapter 5

Applying to College

Applying to college may seem intimidating. But with the right timing, organization, and know-how, it can be a very rewarding process. Let's walk through the application process by going through some of the most common questions about applying to college.

When Should I Start Exploring Colleges?

The earlier the better. There is no such thing as exploring colleges too soon. During freshman and sophomore years, you should already have a list of schools in which you are interested. Start by exploring online. Most universities will provide the important information on their websites: average GPA, average SAT/ACT, tuition, testing requirements, and so forth. Don't eliminate a college based solely on tuition, as it may be able to provide you with scholarships or financial assistance. And remember that the average GPA and SAT scores are just that…an average. Half of the students would have scored lower than the average. So don't rule out schools because your scores don't hit their averages.

When Should I Start to Apply?

The answer here is the same…early! You should start putting together your college application in late summer between your junior and senior years, with the plan to submit your application early in the fall. Many institutions have rolling admissions. In other words they start accepting students just as soon as applications start coming in. As spots get filled, it can become harder and harder for late applicants to get accepted. Applying early is always to your advantage. Your application should be ready to submit the very first day that they are accepting applications! This strategy also means getting your letters of recommendation in time. Be sure to give your teachers at least two to three weeks to write your letters and specify up front the date you need them.

A good approach is to say, "I would need this recommendation by [insert date]. Will that be okay?" It is okay to remind the person gently when the deadline approaches.

How Do I Apply?

The application process starts with reviewing the admissions website for each potential school. Many schools use the Common Application, which allows you to fill out one central application and send it to multiple colleges. Some schools that use the Common Application will also ask for a Common Application Supplement with additional questions that are not present on the Common Application. In addition to individual college websites, you can visit www.commonapp.org to determine if your schools of interest accept the Common Application. If the school doesn't use it, many still accept their individual applications online. You can request materials about the college from their website as well.

Where Do I Apply?

Many factors will go into this decision. Some factors to consider are location, college size, tuition, offered curriculum, social scene, and whether the institution offers extracurriculars that interest you. Beginning to narrow down your schools of interest before you apply is to your advantage. The application process can be time-consuming and expensive. Each school charges a nonrefundable application fee, although waivers are possible if you show financial need. See chapter 7 for more information on selecting the right school for you.

Chapter 6

Funding for College

The average cost of tuition and fees for only one year at a four-year university in 2017–2018 was $9,528 for an in-state public school, $21,632 for an out-of-state public school, and $34,699 for a private school (source: U.S. News and World Report). Unfortunately it is not getting any cheaper. Many high school students ignore the financial aspects and simply try to go to the best school they possibly can. After all, if you go to a great school, you will get a great job and have plenty of money to pay off this debt, right? *Wrong!* Student debt can hang over you for many decades after you finish school. It is important to realize this in high school.

You want to set yourself up for financial success in the future, and step one is to avoid putting yourself in a hole before you even have a job. Although many start off college with the aspiration of becoming a doctor or other well-paying occupation, many people will also change their minds during college for one reason or another. Even those who become doctors hit the sad realization that they will be earning very little until they are out of residency, which is typically in your thirties, and even then most doctors do not make the kind of money they once did. Don't be naïve. Plan early.

The best way to ensure your financial future is a bright one is to minimize student loans. If you don't have the luxury of having rich parents, this can be done through scholarships and need-based financial aid. Let's talk first about scholarships.

Scholarships are typically merit-based awards given to qualified students that they do not have to pay back. One great source for information on scholarships is directly through the schools to which you are applying because many have their own scholarship programs. Another great source is your high school's guidance counselor. They typically are aware of the legitimate scholarship opportunities and should be receiving regular announcements regarding application deadlines and instructions. Third, check to see if the company your parents work for or your local religious institution sponsors a scholarship program.

Some websites are dedicated to providing lists of scholarships. These are worth joining, but I would still recommend that your primary source be your guidance counselor and the admission's office of colleges to which you are applying. Websites for scholarships often flood you with so many possible opportunities that it can be difficult to sift through which ones are legitimate. The websites can be useful for finding opportunities that are not well known and might apply to your unique situation, such as scholarships based on ethnic background, religious affiliation, or military status. Some of these websites are listed at the end of this chapter.

The second source of money is through need-based grants and loans. The difference between the two is that grants don't typically require repayment. The federal government and private institutions have a pool of money with which to award grants and loans to those in need. Applying for this pool involves filling out one or two forms. The Free Application for Federal Student Aid (FAFSA) is a form that predominantly determines eligibility for federal aid, while the CSS Profile form is used by universities to give out need-based awards from their own institutions. Again, check the school's website for more information on requirements, additional forms, and time table for applying.

See chapter 38 for more information on planning for a bright financial future.

Websites with scholarship searches:

www.studentaid.ed.gov

www.collegeboard.org

www.fastweb.com

www.scholarships.com

Websites for financial aid applications:

www.fafsa.gov: Allows you to fill out and submit your FAFSA form.

https://cssprofile.collegeboard.org: Official website for filling out the CSS Profile form.

Chapter 7

Choosing the Right School

Your time in college will likely be some of the best years of your life. But in addition to the fun and excitement that comes with independent living, college will also be your springboard into the rest of your professional career. Choosing the right institution is vital. Here are some factors to consider.

Academic Reputation

Many students simply go to the most reputable school to which they are accepted. No doubt this will lead to the most rigorous academic training as well as prestige, but you ought to reconsider this approach. As mentioned before, looking at the financial aspects of these institutions when making your decision is vital. You also need to understand that although a school has a great reputation, this does not guarantee future success. In fact you will likely be surrounded by other academically gifted students in all of your classes, making it more challenging to get top scores in every class. You must balance the possibility of a lower overall GPA at a more prestigious college with the mere fact that it is prestigious. I am by no means trying to dissuade you from attending a top college. In fact I encourage you to shoot for the best. However, realize that a high ranking by some magazine does not make it the right place for you.

Location

Staying in-state is attractive for many students because it will often provide for a much cheaper tuition to public universities and maintain closeness to family and friends. That being said, it can also involve surprise visits from parents and slightly less independence. Safety of the campus and surrounding community is an important consideration for many, especially if you plan to live off campus. Weather can also greatly affect your college experiences.

Tuition and Finances

Don't rule out any school until you have a complete picture of scholarships, grants, and financial aid that will be offered. This complete picture typically develops near the end of the process when it is time to make a decision. Frank discussion about what your parents can afford to contribute—if anything—is also important.

The "Feeling"

Many students will claim that when they toured a certain college, they just knew they belonged there. They had a "feeling" that this was the place for them. I encourage everyone to visit campuses, talk to current students, and take tours. Hopefully one of your colleges will stick out in your mind as the place that just feels right.

This concludes the high school section. I hope the advice helps put you on the path to success.

Section II
College

This section is dedicated to helping you get started on your journey to medical school. It starts with the raw numbers: How many people apply? How many are accepted? What are the average GPA and MCAT scores of those accepted? It then helps determine if medical school is right for you by presenting an honest look at what medical school entails. The section concludes with advice on the various steps toward a successful application to medical school.

Chapter 8

The Numbers Behind Medical School

Let's start with the basics. At the time of writing this book, there were a total of 141 accredited allopathic medical schools and thirty-three accredited osteopathic medical schools within the United States. For a list of these schools, please see appendices B and C. What are your chances of getting into medical school? To help answer this, here are the important numbers behind the application process. All data come from the American Association of Medical Colleges (AAMC). The following data were collected from 2016 to 2018.

Total number of applicants to medical school: 53,042

Total number that enrolled into medical school: 21,030

Average total GPA for all applicants: 3.55

Average total GPA for those enrolled: 3.70

Average science GPA for all applicants: 3.45

Average science GPA for those enrolled: 3.64

Average MCAT Score for all applicants: 501.8

Average MCAT Score for those enrolled: 508.7

The following are the acceptance rates for applicants based solely on MCAT scores. Data are combined from 2016-2018.

MCAT Score	Acceptance Rate (%)
Less than 486	0.5
486-489	1.3
490-493	3.6
494-497	11.3
498-501	22.3
502-505	35.8
506-509	49.7
510-513	63.7
514-517	75.3
Greater than 517	84.2

The following are acceptance rates for applicants based solely on GPA. Data are from 2016-2018.

GPA	Acceptance Rate (%)
Less than 2.00	3.2
2.00–2.19	0.0
2.20–2.39	4.7
2.40–2.59	5.3
2.60–2.79	6.1
2.80–2.99	9.5
3.00–3.19	15.2
3.20–3.39	22.2
3.40–3.59	32.5
3.60–3.79	48.2
Greater than 3.79	67.1

The following are the acceptance rates for applicants based on their ethnicity. Data are from 2017-2018.

Ethnicity	Acceptance Rate (%)
Black or African American	35
Asian	43
Hispanic or Latino	41
White	44

For more charts and further breakdown of percentages, I encourage you to visit the AAMC website (www.aamc.org/data/facts). The numbers are sliced and diced in every way imaginable.

I hope this helps give you a sense of your chances of acceptance. Depending on your GPA and MCAT scores, these numbers might be frightening or uplifting. In one sense you can see that there is no such thing as a guaranteed admission, but at the same time, almost any applicant can afford some amount of hope. For those who have great grades and are now frightened by the fact that only 67.1% of those with a GPA above 3.8 end up getting accepted, don't be. In my experience, not getting accepted to medical schools despite having great grades is usually due to poor MCAT score, the applicant getting cocky and only applying to top schools, or because the applicant has other problems on his/her personal record that make the candidate undesirable.

Please *do not* get fixated on these numbers. You should simply attempt to do your absolute best in school and let the cards fall where they may.

Chapter 9

Medical School—What's It Really Like?

You're trying to decide if medical school is right for you, but you don't have a good grasp of what's ahead, right? This section will give you a better sense of your future should you choose to become a doctor.

The traditional allopathic medical school in the United States is a four-year commitment. Typically the first two years are dedicated to the basic science of medicine through lecture-based learning in the classroom, while the latter two years are spent in the hospital learning clinical medicine by working alongside doctors.

The first two years involve a high volume of material in a variety of courses. The exact courses may vary among medical schools. These classes help establish the basic science foundation necessary to practice medicine. For more details regarding courses and format, see chapter 22.

During these first two years, most schools attempt to expose students to actual patient care and have courses dedicated to the intangible aspects of medicine, such as learning to take a history and perform a physical, establish rapport with patients, deliver bad news, and so forth. Some time may also be dedicated to working alongside a doctor in clinics. Students are typically just shadowing physicians as opposed to making any decisions in patient care at this point.

The atmosphere during these two initial years can vary quite a bit. Each student tackles them differently. The most important variable is you. For the most part, the structure is similar to college in that you attend classes with your peers, take exams, and spend much of your free time studying. Classes may range from only half a day to a full day. You may have labs for courses like gross anatomy and pathology in which you work with actual anatomy specimens.

The most notable change from the college experience is the sheer volume of material covered. Topics in medical school are covered quickly. Nothing is necessarily complicated about the material itself; it's the quantity. Students typically leave themselves enough time to memorize as much as they can prior to the test only to unlearn everything immediately after and start the process of memorizing again for the next exam. It is a poor method for learning, and most medical school graduates cannot recall much of what they learned during these two years of medical school. But the core concepts stick!

The grading system varies among schools. Some use the A–F standard, while others only grade pass/fail. Some use honors/pass/fail as a way to highlight those students who perform particularly well during these courses.

I mentioned the most important variable during these years is you, and this is why. Some students are quite satisfied with simply making it into medical school and work just enough to get by with every examination. They feel that as long as they pass, they will earn their MD. They tend to be much less stressed and uptight than the regular medical student. On the other hand, some are incredibly preoccupied with grades and feel that anything short of the best grade is a failure. The A–F grading system tends to be much more stressful for these types of students given the constant desire for an A. The vast majority of students fall somewhere in between, and it's those who find a nice balance between studying and living life who are happier and healthier. In chapter 39 I give advice on dealing with the workload and stress.

The third year of medical school takes the students out of the comfortable classroom and puts them into the hospital as they work with various teams of doctors in a variety of specialties. The year usually covers the core rotations, which consist of internal medicine, surgery, pediatrics, obstetrics and gynecology, psychiatry, neurology, and family medicine. Students will have outpatient experiences in which they work in clinic settings. However, the majority of time is spent doing work on the inpatient side, which consists of patients who have been admitted to the hospital due to serious illness for further evaluation and treatment. During the inpatient time, you work in a team that consists of an attending (the main doctor who makes the final decision on patient care), the resident doctor (a medical school graduate who is completing residency in a particular specialty), and the intern (the name given to someone in the first year of residency).

The third year of medical school tends to be the biggest transition for most students and also the most stressful. It is a less structured environment than lecture learning, and this scenario often leads to uneasiness about the role, self-doubt about performance, and worry over evaluations. It can also be nerve-racking when students have to present patients to the team during rounds. The days can also be quiet long, with many rotations requiring students to arrive as early as six o'clock in the morning (or perhaps even earlier). Some rotations expect students to stay overnight for a handful of days during the rotation. Despite its challenges this is often when students first begin to feel like doctors!

Let's go through a typical day on the inpatient side. First you are assigned a few patients (usually no more than three). In the morning you are responsible for examining these patients, getting results for lab values and radiology studies, determining overnight events, and coming up with a preliminary plan for the day. This process is called "prerounding." This can last anywhere from twenty minutes to a few hours depending on the number of patients and the complexity of their medical problems. Residents will often also see the same patients as the students and should know the data on every patient regardless of whether a student is assigned to the patient or not. In essence you, as a student, are there to practice being a resident, but rarely are you given true responsibility over the care and well-being of the patient because you would not yet have the clinical knowledge and experience to make decisions.

The second part of the morning is called "rounds," which involves the entire team working together, including the attending, resident, intern, and medical students. During rounds the team comes up with a formal plan for each patient. This may be done while sitting around a table or more commonly by visiting each patient's room. Rounds typically last a good portion of the morning. The residents and attendings may ask questions of the medical students through rounds to test their knowledge, a process commonly referred to as "pimping." After rounds the remainder of the day is spent helping the resident perform the various tasks that were discussed as a part of rounds. More labs may need to be checked, daily progress notes written, X-rays ordered, patients discharged, and new patients admitted. Often a didactic lecture takes place at noon. Students typically leave the hospital around five or six in the evening, but you may be asked to stay later or even overnight in special situations.

The fourth year is dedicated mostly to elective rotations. As a student, you are allowed to pick rotations that you find interesting. You must also complete at least one rotation in your particular field of interest. During this rotation you are given more responsibility over patient care than during the third year. This rotation is referred to as a subinternship (sub-I) or acting internship (AI) because you, the student, should try to fulfill the role of an intern. Overall because the majority of the fourth year is filled with elective rotations, this year tends to be less stressful and less demanding than is third year. The last few months of medical school are notorious for being the least productive few months, as most students already know where they will be going for residency and lose some motivation to perform at their best. It's the medical school version of "senioritis."

The atmosphere during these latter two years will often vary depending on your personality. Those who are more socially adept tend to find these years easier as they bond with patients and other members of the health care team. Those who are slightly more reserved tend to find the transition to clinical medicine more anxiety provoking. Everyone will run into a resident or attending during this time who they find confrontational or disagreeable. It's an unfortunate part of the learning process in a system that is filled with hierarchies. As a medical student, you are at the bottom of the totem pole, and someone may feel the need to make sure you know this. Others are just angry at life due to their workload and personal problems, and therefore they are not pleasant to work with. Thankfully the majority of residents, nurses, and attendings you encounter this year should be dedicated to helping you advance your medical education. The last two years of medical school are discussed further in chapter 27.

I hope this provides you with a better sense of how medical school is organized and what you may encounter during your years of school. Although the organization I've described for the curriculum is the typical structure, realize that this varies greatly. For example at the Duke

University School of Medicine, there is one year of basic science courses, clinic rotations during second year, an entire year dedicated to research or another degree during third year, and then rotations again during fourth year. Medical schools should provide an overview of their curriculum during the interview process. It's also typically described on their websites.

Overall the four years of medical school are challenging and filled with new experiences and discovery. Each person experiences this differently. Living in a new city, having more work than ever before, and spending less time with family and friends can be difficult. But with a positive attitude and a healthy balance between work and play, these four years can be some of the most productive and rewarding years of your life.

Chapter 10

Is Medical School Right for You?

The question is a tough one, but one that is always important to ask. I encourage anyone interested in medical school to continue to think of other options for themselves and investigate those options as they explore medicine. Convince yourself that medicine is your calling. Don't do it because it's the competitive or prestigious avenue to take. Don't convince yourself you will be rich as a doctor. Most importantly, don't go into medicine because others want you to. Self-motivation is your biggest ally during medical training, which is a long and arduous process. The field of medicine is also one that is constantly changing, so it is important that you are flexible and interested in being a lifelong learner. If you fulfill the following checklist, medicine may be for you:

- ☐ You enjoy helping others.
- ☐ Going into medicine is a decision you have made, not one that others have made for you.
- ☐ You understand that medicine is not the road to riches, but typically a road to a financially comfortable life.

☐ You feel that some sacrifice of time and energy during your training and your future career is acceptable.

☐ You are comfortable being a lifelong learner.

Please keep in mind that when you are going through residency, one of the most difficult times of your training, many of your friends who chose other careers will already be done with school and making higher wages than you while working fewer hours. You have to keep the end goal in sight and not get frustrated by this. Medical training is delayed gratification at its best. I don't say all of this to discourage you but merely to introduce a reality check. I love what I do. I enjoyed the road, and I can't imagine doing anything else. But at the same time, many are unhappy with their decision and regret going into medicine. I don't want you to be one of those people. Hopefully this chapter has not only challenged your decision to pursue medicine, but also reaffirmed it.

Chapter 11

Accelerated Programs and DO Programs

Now that you're convinced that medicine is for you, let's explore some of the options for becoming a doctor.

Accelerated Premed/Medical Programs

A variety of programs throughout the United States offer high school students the option of applying to a joint undergraduate/medical school program. Essentially it is meant to guarantee admission to medical school straight out of high school. Depending on how the program is organized, it may offer an early graduation from undergraduate training after two or three years. For those in high school, such programs represent attractive options. However, you must understand the advantages and disadvantages before you decide if such a program is right for you.

First the advantages. The obvious advantage is being guaranteed a spot in medical school, which may prevent a great deal of stress and anxiety during the undergraduate years. The other advantage is shortening your overall years in school, which is a big financial incentive, as you avoid an extra year or two of tuition. Given the length of medical training, shaving years whenever possible is also nice so that you are a full-fledged doctor earlier in your life.

However, there are quite a few disadvantages. First, although I said "guaranteed spot in medical school" in the prior paragraph, this is often not the case. As an undergraduate, you would typically be required to maintain a certain GPA and also obtain a certain score on the MCAT before being accepted into the medical school. These requirements range quite a bit depending on the school, and you need to know what is expected of you prior to applying. Second, if the program cuts a year or two off of undergraduate time, this is because you will typically be working through the summers and maintaining a vigorous workload. This route can take away from your social life and college experience. Third, if you are smart enough to be accepted into an accelerated program, it is quite possible that you would have been a candidate for a more prestigious medical school had you avoided the combined program. Finally, and perhaps most importantly, high school students rarely have any idea what a life in medicine entails or what they really want in life. Medicine is usually viewed as the most competitive thing to do, thus driving their desire to become doctors. Half of the students at my undergraduate institution reported they were interested in medicine when they started. This number drops off very rapidly.

If you want my advice, I would say be weary of the joint undergraduate/medical school programs. Allow yourself the time to enjoy and experience college. Keep yourself open to any and all career options while you are young. Remember that if you are smart enough to get into these joint programs as a high school student, chances are you will do very well taking the traditional route by going to a regular undergraduate school, taking the MCAT, and then applying to medical schools. You may end up at a better medical school than if you had applied to the combined programs out of high school. Or you may decide that medicine is not for you.

Allopathic versus Osteopathic schools

If you've read this far and still think medicine is your calling, let's talk about the options. You may often hear the terms allopathic and osteopathic when talking about medical schools. What are these exactly, and what is the difference between the two?

Allopathic medical schools result in an MD degree, which is the more common degree for medical physicians. Osteopathic medical schools award a DO degree. They are both legally equivalent. DO degree holders can practice medicine in the exact same way as an MD. However, the DO curriculum puts more emphasis on patients as a whole with the belief that the body must be treated as a whole to get better. The DO curriculum also has a class in osteopathic manipulative medicine (OMM), which uses manipulation of the musculoskeletal system to treat various medical conditions. Apart from that the curriculums are very similar. They both pursue residencies after medical school. A larger percentage of DO degree holders go into primary care than do MD degree holders.

Many believe that the MD degree is the more prestigious of the two, as the average MCAT and GPA scores tend to be higher for acceptance to an allopathic school than for an osteopathic school. The MD degree also tends to be more readily identified to denote a "doctor" by the general public. However, this perception is slowly changing, and the distinction between MD and DO is becoming less obvious as awareness of DO schools grows. I know many DO degree holders who work in my hospital, and they are great clinicians. If DO school is something you might be interested in, please visit aacom.org for further information. For a list of allopathic and osteopathic medical schools in the United States, please see appendices B and C.

Chapter 12

Premedical Prerequisites

Most medical schools in the United States have similar sets of prerequisites that students must fulfill prior to applying. For undergraduate coursework it typically includes the following:

One year of biology

Two years of chemistry (including organic chemistry)

One year of physics

One year of English

A few schools also require biochemistry, but most do not. Some also ask for more than one year of biology. It is very important to start researching medical schools early in your undergraduate years. I advise students to start their research at the beginning of their sophomore year to determine if their schools of interest have biochemistry as a prerequisite.

In addition to coursework, most medical schools also require applicants to take the Medical College Admission Test (MCAT). Please see chapter 15 for tips on taking the MCAT.

Apart from the prerequisites, as a student, you are allowed to study and major in any subject. This concept brings us to our next chapter.

Chapter 13

What Should I Major In?

This question comes up often. As you've seen in the prior chapter, the prerequisites for coursework are not overly cumbersome. Students who apply to medical school can major in any subject they choose so long as those prerequisites are also completed.

But is there a major (or double major) that makes you a more attractive applicant to medical schools? My answer would be no. My advice for choosing a major is to select one that you will enjoy learning about and one in which you will do well. Of course choosing a very unchallenging major will look questionable, but so long as it is a respectable major, the choice is yours. You should not choose biochemistry for the sole reason of trying to impress medical schools if you do not like biochemistry. Chances are, your grades will reflect your lack of interest, and you will end up being a less attractive applicant to medical school.

In my medical school class, half of the students were non-science majors as undergraduates. So don't put too much pressure on yourself to choose the right major because there isn't one!

For those who want the numbers, here is a chart that breaks it all down. The bottom line is that all majors have roughly the same acceptance rate. Do what you enjoy!

Undergrad Major	Number of Applicants	Number Enrolled in Medical School	Approximate Acceptance Rate (%)
Biological Sciences	27,653	10,675	39
Humanities	2,160	1,057	49
Math and Statistics	438	192	44
Physical Sciences	5,102	2,319	45
Social Sciences	5,629	2,277	40

Source: American Association of Medical Colleges

Chapter 14

Tips for the Application

The two most important factors in medical school admissions are your GPA and MCAT scores. They form the foundation on which the rest of your application is built. Medical schools have to set certain criteria to narrow down the thousands of applications they receive, so these scores typically serve as the initial screen.

The most important advice I can give you regarding your GPA is to get focused early. Undergraduate courses are much harder than high school. Even if you were the child prodigy and star of your local town, you will have to work hard in college. Remember this from the very beginning, and start college with a strong GPA.

Do not fall into the trap of thinking, "Ah, I'll just pull up my GPA later." A low GPA becomes *very* hard to pull up; start strong.

Although GPA and MCAT scores set the stage, much more is involved in getting accepted. The application to medical school also asks for a personal statement, work/activities, and letters of reference. Let's discuss each of these.

The personal statement is an essay written by each applicant that addresses an open-ended question, such as, "Why have you decided to pursue a career in medicine?" The appropriate length for your personal statement is typically about one single-spaced page. You do not have to fill the entire space allotted. More is not necessarily better. The personal statement should also be just that...personal. It should be about your journey and the reasons behind your passion for the field. It is often advised to start out the personal statement with something that immediately gets the reader's attention. Remember that the admissions committee members have to read hundreds of these essays. Try to keep them engaged and entertained. Start working on your personal statement early. After you have completed a first draft, take a break from it for a few days and then come back and read it again. This makes awkward sentences stand out. If you are working on the essay nonstop for multiple days, spotting these sentences may be hard because you become too close to the work. I also recommend you have others read it, such as family members or even faculty members you know well. For grammar start by reading the last sentence of the essay and work your way up, as this method makes it easier to spot errors.

Every application will also ask about your work experience/activities. Being a well-rounded applicant is very important. Having only a great GPA and MCAT may get your foot in the door for an interview, but having a solid application with a variety of extracurricular activities helps seal the deal.

These activities can be anything you think medical schools will find worthwhile. They should include some activities related to the medical field, but I highly encourage students to participate in nonmedical activities as well. Volunteer organizations, sports teams, and student government are just a few examples. Many people ask whether it is necessary to shadow a doctor. Personally I don't feel that shadowing should be a major activity. If the only thing you are doing is following a doctor around all day, you haven't really contributed anything. Shadowing is more of an activity for you. It's a way for you to get a better sense of what medicine entails. Some would disagree with this opinion. It is fine to include it on your application, but please don't spend a hundred hours shadowing and expect admissions committees to be impressed. They know what shadowing involves, and once again, more is not necessarily better. Spending a few days shadowing might be more than enough.

Remember to participate in a variety of activities, not just one or two. On the 2018 American Medical College Application System (AMCAS) application, there were fifteen available spaces to enter work, activities, honors/awards, and publications on the primary medical school application. Although quality involvement is very important, quantity typically catches the eye easier (even if it seems unfair to those who spend many hours in one activity). To help acknowledge which activities required more time commitment, the application also asks you to estimate the total number of hours you spent involved with the activity. You can highlight up to three activities as the "most meaningful" and then describe these activities further.

If your school allows you to participate in research with a faculty member, consider getting involved. It is one activity that tends to stand out on an application. Also with every activity, keep a record of your supervisor as well as the person's contact number or e-mail address. The initial application to medical school will ask you to list this information in case they want to call and verify the work you did. I imagine they actually use this contact information very rarely. But if there is an application that raises suspicion for falsifying information, I'm sure they would not hesitate to make some calls.

Finally, letters of reference play an important role in a well-rounded application. Ask for these letters well before you think you will need them. Most professors are incredibly busy. You don't want their schedules to be the reason your application gets turned in late. Always ask early! Give them at least one month, but more is better.

As far as choosing from whom to get reference letters, the key is finding someone who knows you well. That might be difficult if all of your classes had two hundred people. Make an effort to get to know a few professors. Visit them during office hours, work hard in their courses, and speak up in class. If you do participate in undergraduate research and it goes well, ask your advisor for a letter. Don't be ashamed to ask your professors if they feel they can write you a *strong* letter of recommendation. If you get a hesitant answer, best to ask someone else. And although it looks great to have a letter from the chair of some department, remember that if they don't know you well, the letter will likely be a weak one. It's better to get a strong letter from a junior faculty member rather than a weak one from the chair.

Chapter 15

Tips for the MCAT

Acing the MCAT is much like acing any other test. The key is solid preparation and knowledge of the exam content with frequent practice. My recommendation is to take a preparatory course. Having an instructor go over the material is helpful, but for me, an important part was the reading material the course provided. I made it my goal to learn every miniscule detail in those books.

But perhaps the most important part about taking a course was access to countless practice questions. This was where I really had to apply what I learned. The MCAT is not a test of just rote memorization and recall. Doing well takes practice and the ability to apply the concepts you learned to different situations. Courses like Kaplan and Princeton Review will also administer multiple full-length practice exams leading up to the real thing. Practice, practice, practice! Many people hesitate to take courses given the expense. If the expense makes the course unfeasible, find a solid independent study guide. My followers often recommend the Examkrackers study materials.

In the few weeks leading up to the test, start getting to sleep a bit earlier. If you are up routinely until midnight every night studying, falling asleep early the night before the test will be impossible. Start waking up early as well and work on practice problems as soon as you awaken. Get accustomed to using your brain early in the morning. Having your sleep cycle and circadian rhythm in the right spot will help keep you focused and alert during the exam.

On the day prior to the exam, try to take it easy. Ideally do not study; just relax and get some rest. I do recommend checking out the exam location before the test date. Try driving there at the same time you would on the real day to get a sense of traffic and how long it will take you. Give yourself plenty of extra time to get to the test site. The last thing you want before the MCAT is a stressful ride to the test center.

For more information on test overview, material tested, registration, and so forth, visit www.aamc.org/mcat.

Chapter 16

The Application Process

The process of applying to medical school starts in early summer one year prior to the start of medical school. Almost all medical schools in the United States start the application process with the American Medical College Application Service (AMCAS), which is organized by the Association of American Medical Colleges (AAMC). The exception at the time of writing this book includes many of the public MD programs in Texas. The online AMCAS application typically opens in May for students to begin filling out, but allows students to submit their applications roughly one month later. Deadlines for individual schools vary but are typically between October and December. Please start filling this application out *as soon as possible*!

The following are the components of the AMCAS application:

Section 1, 2, and 3: Demographic information

Section 4: Coursework

Section 5: Work experience, extracurricular activities, awards, etc. (15 spots available, can pick up to three activities to describe in further detail)

Section 6: Evaluation Letters

Section 7: List of medical schools to which you are applying

Section 8: Personal statement (5300 character limit, including spaces)

Section 9: MCAT scores (automatically released to AMCAS)

I highly recommend having this application completed and ready to send on the first day the application is allowed to be submitted. Many medical schools admit students based on rolling admissions. They start accepting students right after their first round of interviews. Typically as spots fill up, getting a remaining spot becomes a bit more challenging. You want to be one of the first applicants and interviewees at these institutions.

Once your AMCAS application is complete, you will be allowed to designate which schools should receive this preliminary application. Then you wait as the schools screen these preliminary applications and send most students who applied a secondary (aka supplemental) application. Each school has a different secondary application, with a wide range of additional information it will want. Schools often have short essay questions with very specific topics. Again the key is to fill out the applications expeditiously, yet thoughtfully, and return them to the schools. Please make sure that all of your applications are free of spelling errors. In medicine, details matter. You don't want to show medical schools that you aren't paying attention to the details.

Once the secondary application is submitted, the applications are again screened by the schools. Those who make the second round of cuts are invited to interview. If all goes well during the interview, you will hopefully get that long-awaited letter in the mail accepting you to the medical school of your dreams.

Chapter 17

Interviewing

The following is a list of my top tips for a successful medical school interview. For those of you who have read my book *Why Medicine? And 500 Other Questions for the Medical School and Residency Interview*, these may sound familiar.

Tip 1: Know your application

You will quickly discover that the majority of questions will be about your application. This works in your favor because you should know your application better than anyone else. Always keep a copy of the application with you, and review it the night before your interview. Recall the type of work you did for each extracurricular activity. This is especially true for research. Never be caught saying, "I only cleaned the test tubes." Even if you just did manual labor, you should know the type of research the laboratory performed and its goals. Not knowing the details behind your activities is a major red flag and tells the interviewer that you participated superficially just to write it on your resume.

Tip 2: Know the location

I made it a habit to drive to the hospital the night before my interview so I knew exactly where I was going. Knowing the directions takes one stress away from what will already be a stressful day. Never trust Google Maps or your GPS. See it for yourself!

Tip 3: Time should be on your side

Nothing gets the interview day off to a worse start than running late. It creates stress for you, and if you do show up late, it hurts your chances of acceptance. Instead, plan to get there thirty minutes earlier than scheduled. If you are there early, walk around or read over your application. Time should be your friend during the interview process.

Tip 4: Dress the part

The interview trail is not the place to experiment with the latest in fashion. Stick with the convention. For women, a suit is the norm, with the skirt suit being the most common. A pantsuit is perfectly acceptable. If you go with a skirt, make sure it is the appropriate length (at least to the knees). For men, a suit is a must. The colors for men and women are similar. Stick with navy blue, black, or gray. Avoid excessive perfume or cologne. They should remember you for what you said and not how you smelled.

Tip 5: Keep talking

The key to a successful interview is staying loose. I forced myself to make conversation with my fellow interviewees and talked about neutral topics that had nothing to do with the interview process. This was a great way to stay relaxed. Sitting in a corner by yourself and thinking about the upcoming interview may have the opposite effect.

Tip 6: Be honest

You have probably heard this advice countless times. The best way to ruin your chances of being offered a spot in a program is to lie. In addition nothing gets you more nervous during an interview than stretching the truth—not to mention that you are about to embark on a career path where your integrity and character mean everything. Stick with the truth.

What will they ask during the interview? Anything is fair game, but typically questions will come directly from your application because interviewers want to discuss your prior extracurriculars and experiences. Here are a few common questions. For a complete list of more than five hundred common interview questions, I would encourage you to read my book *Why Medicine? And 500 Other Questions for the Medical School and Residency*

Interview. Preparing for interviews is important, and knowing the right questions to think about will help you ace the interview.

1. Why do you want to go into medicine?
2. What got you interested in our institution?
3. What are you looking for in a medical school?
4. Do you think our institution is a good fit for you?
5. What makes you stand out from the other applicants?
6. Tell me about ____ (fill in the blank with one of your activities).
7. Which extracurricular activity are you most proud of?
8. Which activities got you interested in medicine?
9. What would you do if you couldn't go into medicine?
10. What are your strengths and weaknesses?
11. How would your friends describe you?
12. Where do you see yourself in ten years?
13. What is your favorite book?
14. Tell me about a time you took on a leadership role.
15. A life in medicine means a life of service to others. How have you shown your dedication to serving others?

16. What characteristics would you want in your doctor?
17. What characteristics will make you a good doctor?
18. Do you know what type of doctor you want to be?
19. What challenges do you foresee in your future as a doctor?
20. Do you have any questions for me? (Always have a question ready)

Chapter 18

Applying to US Schools for Foreign Students

According to the AAMC, in 2017 there were 1,933 foreign applicants to US medical schools, of which 350 were accepted and 274 matriculated into a US medical school. In 2018 only forty-nine schools reported that they even accepted applications from international students. As you can see, admission for a foreign student to a US medical school is challenging, but not impossible. Check with individual schools to determine if they accept international applications. Most schools will require international students to complete some coursework in the US, particularly if the coursework from their college abroad is not recognized by US schools.

The application process itself is fairly similar. Students are required to apply through the AMCAS application. International coursework is not recognized through this application unless it is verified and credited through an undergraduate school in the United States. The last barrier for international students is funding their educations. Unfortunately international students are not eligible for many government-funded loan programs. Schools often ask for proof of funds to cover tuition, or they may even ask for all four years of expenses to be paid up front. For further information please refer to this one-page summary published by the AAMC (https://goo.gl/K18NRB). Here you will find additional links for further information.

Chapter 19

Choosing a Medical School

If you are lucky enough to be accepted to multiple medical schools, you now have the task of picking where you want to spend the next four years. Allow me to give you a few factors to take into consideration before you make your final decision.

First, money matters. Don't be fooled into thinking you will be rich once you finish your medical training and that paying back loans will be a cinch. The fact of the matter is that physicians are not compensated nearly as well as most would believe. No doubt the life of a physician overall is quite comfortable, but comfortable is far from rich. Consider how much you may already owe in loans from your undergraduate education, and think twice before signing up for another heap of loans. Consider a public in-state school if that tuition looks favorable. Most accredited medical schools in the United States will provide you with the necessary education to become a competent doctor, so don't force yourself into a situation you won't be able to afford. Your loans will follow you for many years after completing training, so plan accordingly.

71

Please see chapter 38 for further guidance on financial matters.

Second, something is to be said about your gut feeling. At which school did you feel most comfortable, got along well with faculty, and noticed a happy group of students? Which geographic area naturally appeals to you? Where will you enjoy spending the next four years? Medical school is a tough time, but being among a group that you mesh with and feel secure around helps.

Third, if you fall within the minority of students who already know what field you want to pursue before entering college, this could factor into your choice as well. If you are focused on pursuing a primary-care field such as family medicine or pediatrics, perhaps you will be better suited at a public school that focuses on producing primary-care practitioners for its state. If you want to be a neurosurgeon that specializes in the spine, then it might be to your advantage to pick a larger, research-oriented medical school that ranks highly so that you are a competitive candidate for such a residency. But remember, no matter which medical school you attend, you can match in any residency you choose so long as you perform well.

Lastly get a sense of which curriculum you will thrive in. I loved the honors/pass/fail system at my medical school. I found it much less stressful than the traditional

A–F system that I had endured for so long. However, some like the added motivation of seeking that "A" and are drawn to grading systems that provide for more stratification in academic performance.

Chapter 20

I Didn't Get In. Now What?

The sad reality is that not everyone is accepted to medical school. It is a competitive process. Of the 51,680 students who applied in 2017, only 21,338 ended up enrolling. So what options are available to those who received no acceptance letters? The first question is this: Will you reapply next year? If the answer is yes, continue reading below. If the answer is no, skip to the next section, "Alternative Career Paths."

For those who plan to reapply, the two main ways to increase your chances of acceptance are to improve your application and apply to a broader range of schools. How can you improve your application? First, call the admission's offices of every school to which you applied and ask if they can provide feedback on how to improve your application. Be polite and not pushy; you will likely be applying there again next year. You might find that certain aspects stick out, such as GPA or MCAT. If GPA is the main issue, some students opt to do a postbaccalaureate program to improve overall GPA. However, be realistic in how much your GPA will improve. If you have a GPA of 3.0 after four years of college, and you take an additional semester with a similar workload that you had in your college semesters, even if you obtain a perfect 4.0 for the semester, your overall GPA will increase to 3.11. Not a big jump. It's fine to pursue this path if you feel necessary, but do the math first for your situation.

If your MCAT score is the problem, retaking the test is an option. But let's discuss a few points to consider before signing back up. First, was there something about the test day that led to your poor performance, such as an illness or major life event? If so, you should retest. If not, will you plan to prepare a different way for a repeat test? Your answer should be yes if you plan to retake. What are your chances of doing better? AAMC data, not surprisingly, shows those who score very low on the first exam are the most likely to increase their score, while those who score the highest are less likely to improve their score.

Try to spend the next year participating in activities that will strengthen your application. Doing a second degree (such as a master's degree in public health) is one option. Some universities offer programs known as special master's programs (SMPs), which may serve as a transition to medical school. Performing a year of research is another option. You will be asked about what you did during this gap year when you interview again. Doing something productive is vital.

The last important consideration when reapplying is to broaden the types of schools to which you apply. You should definitely apply to all of your public in-state schools. If you only applied to MD programs, consider DO programs as well. Some students also look to international programs and Caribbean medical schools. In my experience, training in these programs is hit or miss. You want to ensure their curriculum is properly accredited. Many international schools will offer clinical rotations at American hospitals. I know many students who have gone to the Caribbean medical schools and ended up finding residencies in pediatrics, family medicine, and internal medicine. However, obtaining a residency in the more competitive programs, such as orthopedic surgery and dermatology, may be more difficult no matter how well you do in school if you go to an overseas medical school. Ask about the percentage of students that match into residency after medical school. Some Caribbean schools match less than 50% of their students! Students may also have difficulty passing their board exams after doing medical training in international medical schools, so keep this in mind as well. Graduates from Caribbean medical schools and other international programs fall into the category of foreign medical graduate, or FMG. For detailed information on the application process for FMGs, please refer to www.ecfmg.org.

Alternative Career Paths

If medical school did not work out or you have come to the conclusion that it isn't a good fit for you, but you are still interested in health care and helping others, rest assured that many other careers are out there for you. Some career paths to consider strongly include physician assistant, dentistry, nursing, respiratory therapy, occupational therapy, and physical therapy, to name just a few. Explore your options. Health care involves much more than just being a medical doctor. Here are some resources to begin exploring these fields:

Physician Assistant Education Association
www.paeaonline.org

American Dental Association
www.ada.org/education.aspx

American Association of Colleges of Nursing
www.aacn.nche.edu

American Association for Respiratory Care
www.aarc.org

American Physical Therapy Association

www.apta.org

American Occupational Therapy Association
www.aota.org

This concludes the collegiate portion of this book. Here are some take-home points:

- Go into medicine for you and not anyone else. Self-motivation will be your biggest friend during medical training.
- Focus on starting off college with a strong GPA. Pulling up a low GPA is very hard.
- Choose a major you enjoy and will excel in. Don't pick a major for the sole purpose of impressing a medical school.
- Start preparing for the MCAT early and consider taking a review course. The key to doing well is tons and tons of practice questions.
- DO and MD programs are legally equivalent. Consider DO schools as well in your search.
- Apply to medical school early! Your application should be ready to go on day one.

Dr. K's Checklist for Getting into Medical School

☐ Get into college and maintain a strong GPA.

☐ Prepare early and voraciously for the MCAT.

☐ Participate in a variety of extracurricular activities.

☐ Consider doing a semester of research in a lab.

☐ Fill out the AMCAS application and apply early!

☐ Fill out secondary applications and apply early!

☐ Interview.

☐ Pick a great school.

<u>Section III</u>
Medical School

You've made it! Let's turn you into a medical school star! This section is dedicated to helping you not just survive, but thrive in your new world of medicine.

Chapter 21
Getting Started

Congrats, you are going to be a doctor! Now what? First, enjoy the summer before the start of school. This may be the last time you have such a long vacation with no responsibilities. Avoid the temptation to get a jump-start on the coursework by cracking open a biochemistry textbook. Yes, obsessing over schoolwork has gotten you this far, but starting to learn how to balance life and school is important. Once you are in medicine, the importance of your time and your enjoyment become clear. Don't feel guilty about taking some time to enjoy yourself.

Your official start of medical school will likely take place through a one-week orientation. Use this time to be a social butterfly and get to know your classmates. You will be going through the next four years with these people and will come to rely on them. Start developing a "crew." Find people with whom you will get along, and start trying to socialize with them outside of the hospital. Ask a group to get together for dinner at a popular spot, have people over for a movie, or just go grab a beer. You will find people very willing to socialize and hang out during this initial time, but soon enough, everyone will shuffle out into their own groups. So give yourself a chance to develop a group of core friends. Having friends will help you stay sane through the next four years and perhaps well beyond. But rest assured that even if you don't create a close group, all is not lost. After all, there just isn't as much time to spend with friends as there was in college. Most friends in medical school spend more time studying together than anything else. So being a team of one is okay. In medicine being your own best friend and finding ways to enjoy your time is important, even if it's spent alone. So don't worry if you don't find a group that you mesh with perfectly. I certainly did not. I still enjoyed my medical school years, and so can you.

A bit of advice on relationships. My advice would be to avoid jumping into a romantic relationship with a classmate too early in medical school. Such relationships may isolate you a bit from other classmates, and if things don't work out, you are left without close friends and an awkward relationship with your ex. Take time to develop a core group instead, and if you then find that special someone, great. I've seen plenty of successful relationships and marriages develop in my medical school class, but give it some time.

In the first few weeks, also take some time to explore the city and surrounding area. Figure out what activities you might enjoy during the next four years. Explore now before you get too tied down in the coursework. Find the popular venues for eating and casual nights out. Enjoy your city.

So, in summary…

- Enjoy the summer before entering medical school.
- Develop a core group of friends early; but more importantly, find outlets to enjoy your downtime.
- Avoid jumping into romantic relationships too soon.
- Explore your city.

Chapter 22

The Basic Science Years—The Format

Most medical schools begin with two years of basic science followed by two years of clinical work in the hospital and outpatient clinics. The format for the first two years is similar to high school and college; you sit in a lecture hall, take notes, and take tests.

The first year of courses typically cover the main basic science subjects, such as biochemistry, genetics, cell biology, physiology, anatomy, neurobiology, pathology, immunology, microbiology, pharmacology, and histology. You will also have additional labs, such as gross anatomy (where you dissect human cadavers) and histology (where you look at slides under microscopes). The workload is typically much heavier than during college. However, the material itself is not that difficult. What makes medical school challenging is the volume of work. Knowing every detail about the subject material may have been possible during tests in high school and college, but you will soon find that medical school is a bit different. You may not have time to learn all of the details for every single test. Most students find their own level of comfort as far as preparation for tests. Many are content with just getting by, so they avoid obsessively studying, while others bring their perfectionist tendencies. You have to find your happy middle ground.

During the second year, you continue to learn about the basic sciences, but the material may be reorganized into an organ-based approach. Instead of focusing an entire few weeks on pharmacology and another few weeks on physiology as you did in the first year, you will focus a few weeks on the cardiovascular system or the respiratory system. Alternatively you may learn about all the normal human functions during first year and then focus on pathology during the second. Schools organize these first two years a bit differently, so check their websites for further details. Most programs will incorporate some sort of class that teaches students how to take medical histories from patients, examine them, deliver bad news, and build patient rapport. Typically you will also have some form of patient contact during these two years, such as shadowing a doctor for half a day each week.

Please note that almost all medical schools will tout about how wonderful and recently updated their curriculum is and how it is specifically geared toward creating well-rounded physicians with early patient exposure. It is a common line. At the end of the day, almost all programs are still quite similar. The true exceptions are those programs that do all of the basic science teaching in one year and thus have an extra year during medical school to pursue research or dual degrees. Again check the medical school websites to explore various curriculums.

Helpful Reference Books

Below are suggestions on excellent reference books during your basic science years. Keep in mind that if your medical school recommends a text in particular, using that book is important. This list is based on recommendations from me and hundreds of other medical students.

Biochemistry: *Biochemistry* (Lippincott's Illustrated Review Series) by Denise Ferrier

Cell Biology: *Molecular Biology of the Cell* by Bruce Alberts

Embryology: *High-Yield Embryology* by Ronald Dudek

Genetics: *Thompson & Thompson Genetics in Medicine* by Robert Nussbaum, et al.

Gross Anatomy: *Atlas of Human Anatomy* by Frank Netter (This is just an atlas with pretty pictures. You will need another text to explain the details of anatomy)

Immunology: *The Immune System* by Peter Parham

Microanatomy/Histology: *Histology: A Text and Atlas* by Michael Ross and Wojciech Pawlina

Microbiology: *Microbiology Made Ridiculously Simple* by Mark Gladwin, et al.

Neurobiology: *Neuroscience* by Purves, et al.

Pathology: *Pathologic Basis of Disease* by Vinay Kumar, et al.

Pharmacology: *Pharmacology (Lippincott's Illustrated Review Series)* by Karen Whalen

Physiology: *Guyton and Hall Textbook of Medical Physiology* by John Hall (for more detailed reading), *BRS Physiology* by Linda Costanzo (for fast review)

Chapter 23

Study Strategies for Basic Science Courses

1. My second cousin says how great of a time she had at someone's wedding that I don't know.
2. An old middle school acquaintance comments that his one-year-old child giggles a lot.
3. A college friend wishes her husband a happy birthday.
4. A high school friend comments that there are a lot of "whack celebrities" at some award show I've never heard of.
5. A college acquaintance says she had a great time with great people. She fails to elaborate on who, what, when, where, or why.

I have just read you the last five updates on my Facebook newsfeed. This news, as they call it, tells me nothing, and my life would be no different had I not wasted the last few minutes reading it. And yet somehow I am drawn to Facebook as if I would be missing something if I didn't check my newsfeed every so often. It's the same way I'm drawn to Twitter to check if I have more followers. Sound familiar? If Facebook, Twitter,

Instagram, and Snapchat had been around while I was in high school, I don't think I would have graduated.

The distractions are everywhere. And for the most part, they are quite useless and without substantial information that adds anything to our well-being or furthers our education. These distractions include social media, texts, Netflix, e-mail, and YouTube clips. The list of things that are crying for a short bit of your attention is endless. Collectively I call all of these little distractions "Twextbook." And although individually they might not take up too much of your time, collectively they are a time management disaster! Try to think of the last time you spent over one continuous hour simply focused on studying without any distractions from your own Twextbook. Each time you are distracted, your brain has to completely shift gears to get back on topic; this shift takes time.

After a long day of trying to study while having Twextbook constantly distracting us and making us mind-numbingly inefficient, we have the nerve to say, "Gosh, I just don't have enough time."

The reality that we don't want to admit is that there is plenty of time in the day. Heck, we have the same number of hours in the day that Einstein, Gandhi, and Martin Luther King Jr. had, right? But they didn't have

Twextbook. You do. So my first bit of advice is simple. Let your brain actually spend solid chunks of time (two or three hours) away from Twextbook. Take your notes and your book, and hit the library. Sit in a cubicle so you have nothing to look at other than your books. Turn your cell phone off. Sounds scary, I know, but the world won't implode while you are off the grid for a few hours. If you have to use your laptop to study, do not open up your e-mail in the background. There is no real need to ever check e-mail more than once a day. If something is urgently important, people should find a better way to let you know. If you do all of this and your mind keeps wandering and wanting to check your Instagram feed or urges you to open up Twitter to see what Kim Kardashian is saying, then your brain has become addicted to these little distractions and is no longer trained to focus.

Are you addicted? Try this simple test. Place your phone on your desk while you attempt to read for one continuous hour. No matter how many times your phone vibrates or rings, see if you can make it through one entire hour without looking at it. If this exercise is a struggle for you, or if you find yourself making excuses for why you need to take a quick look, you are an addict. A Twextbook addict. It is your drug, and the first step to treatment is admitting you have a problem.

How do we treat this addiction? Here are five simple steps:

Step 1: Estimate the amount of time you spend each day dedicated to social media, checking e-mail and perusing the web. Be honest.

Step 2: Take that total amount, and divide it into three equal parts. After each meal, take that amount of time to dedicate to Twextbook. Get it out of your system. In between there should be no Twextbooking! Do what it takes, even if this means turning off your phone or leaving your laptop at home while you hit the library. The key to fighting an addiction is not giving in, even when it's difficult.

Step 3: Each week, try to decrease the time you are spending on Twextbook during each of the three chunks by ten minutes. Once you are down to less than twenty minutes per chunk, try to drop one chunk all together, and spend only two times a day dedicated to the distractions.

Step 4: Give yourself a small punishment for when you lapse and check on Twextbook outside of your dedicated chunks. A rubber band on the wrist is one way to do this, giving yourself a self-inflicted flick each time. Make it a little uncomfortable, but not overtly painful. Or take ten minutes out of the next break as punishment.

Step 5: Reward yourself when you are down to less than thirty minutes of distraction time each day by buying yourself something nice.

Doing well in school is partly smarts, but mostly it's about how well you study and your discipline. Plenty of people hit the books without any distractions and soak up the material, so why put yourself at a disadvantage?

Once you've gotten rid of Twextbook, we can move on to my second piece of advice. Having your mind in the right place for studying involves more than avoiding distraction. I learned this a bit too late. In college I convinced myself that I only needed six hours of sleep each night to function. I was wrong. I would fall asleep in every class, and outside of the classroom, I would have my book open for only two minutes before dozing off. As you can imagine, this was inefficiency at its best. More discussion of sleep is in chapter 39, but the bottom line is that the average adult needs seven to nine hours of sleep each night. Most actually need more than eight to feel fully refreshed. You can't change this sleep need; it's genetically determined. So if you keep dozing off during lectures or while studying, it's not because you are bored; it's probably because you don't sleep enough. Being alert throughout the day makes learning much more efficient.

But wait, you say, I'm losing an extra hour or two while sleeping that I could use studying. My rebuttal is that if you are 50 percent more efficient during the day after getting more sleep, who cares if you are studying one or two hours less? You are still learning more, and as an added bonus, you don't feel like you are going to die of exhaustion all the time.

Third, for all tests big or small, try to get a sense of how the test will be structured and what type of questions will be asked. Studying for a multiple-choice test is done differently than studying for open-ended essay questions. For multiple choice you focus more on details and recognition of the right answer rather than pulling the answer from thin air. For open-ended questions, it is important to have a grasp of the bigger picture first and then delve into the details. Make sure you can recall specific words and concepts, not simply recognize them.

Once you have these three basic steps to studying in place, work on some more of the following tips to successful studying:

1. Don't multitask. Studies show we are much worse at multitasking than we think and tend to be much less efficient. Avoid the temptation of trying to clean your room or cook yourself lunch while you study. Focus on one task, get it done, and then move on to the next.

2. Take a short break. Study marathons can be inefficient. Once you feel your brain fighting back and refusing to hold onto study material, take a short break. This is a good time to exercise, eat, or get some sun. Avoid activities that will suck you in and make it hard to get back to the books.

3. Study in short time intervals and repeat. Instead of a long marathon, try to split studying into small sessions to improve retention.

4. Create a scheduled study time each day.

5. Find a dedicated study location.

6. Create a set goal for each study session. For example, get through chapters 1–3 during tonight's session.

7. Read as if you'll have to teach it. This makes the material stick better and forces you to make sense of it.

8. Avoid music. Learning with background music can impair concentration.

9. Study before class. If you've already gone through the material once, class will help solidify the information and give you a chance to ask good questions.

10. Give yourself some extra time. Start studying far enough in advance that you aren't pressured and anxious at the last minute. Plan so that you never have to pull an all-nighter. Having a little bit of stress near test time may actually be a good thing to help you

learn better, but having too much stress will work against you.

To summarize the highlights of this chapter:
- Get rid of any and all distractions when studying.
- Get some sleep. Avoid all-nighters.
- Know what will be tested and how.
- Start studying early for tests and practice good study habits.

Chapter 24

Test-Taking Anxiety

We've all experienced it…you open up the first page of the test, your heart begins racing, you have trouble concentrating, and everything you studied seems to fly out of your brain at just the wrong time. This anxiety is incredibly common and can make even the simplest of tests very uncomfortable. It can be so severe that it causes nausea and vomiting. What's worse, test-taking anxiety is associated with poor performance.

Thankfully there are some easy steps you can take to lessen this anxiety. Here is a list:

1. Get enough sleep. Sleep deprivation can worsen your anxiety.

2. Eat a balanced diet. Getting adequate carbohydrates for a slow release of glucose is important. Think fruits and nuts.

3. Use positive self-imagery. Think of happy images, whatever they may be. Then, right afterward, think about being in your test-taking room. Pairing happy images with your testing environment can lessen anxiety when you arrive.

4. Think of questions you know the answer to just prior to the test. This action will build your confidence.

5. Write down your worries prior to the test. Sometimes unloading these negative thoughts and concerns can help free up your mind during test time.

6. Find an easy question on the test first. Getting through the first question is often the toughest part. Get this first one behind you, and you may find that the anxiety suddenly decreases, allowing you to focus.

Now that you are set up for test-taking success, let's move on to my favorite part of this book—teaching you the ultimate memorization trick!

Chapter 25

The Best Memory Trick Ever!

Get ready to change the way you study. In medical school, much like the rest of education, we rely heavily on rote memorization. It is an unfortunate reality. Testing in school is not typically based on how well we can apply concepts but instead on how much we can memorize and then regurgitate during the examination. In medical school each of my exams was preceded by days of constant cramming. After the test was over, it was as if someone hit the delete button in my head, and *poof*, all the information was gone. Then I was ready to start the process all over again for the next exam.

Let's start off with a test. Set your timer for two minutes, and memorize as many of the words on the next page as you can. Use whatever strategy you typically use to memorize large amounts of material for school. Don't skip over this part; once you learn the new method, it will be hard to go back to your old way of memorizing.

Elephant	Box
George Washington	Chair
Baseball	Gravel
Flamingo	Computer
Apple	Cereal
Hammer	Appendicitis
Telephone	Sweater
Water	Gold
Julia Roberts	Cloud
Freedom	E. coli

Now test yourself by closing the book and listing as many as you can.

How many did you get out of the list of twenty?

In this section I will teach you a trick to make rote memorization much easier. Many of the concepts in this chapter I learned through a memoir called *Moonwalking with Einstein* by Joshua Foer.

My strategy during school was the repetition approach. I'd simply read it again and again and hope it stuck. Most people do this, but it is very inefficient. The reason is that our brains weren't designed to memorize in this way. They were designed to memorize visually.

Close your eyes for a minute and think back to your childhood home, your high school, or even a friend's home you recently visited for the first time. I bet the visual pictures of these places are still fresh in your mind even though you haven't been there in a while or you visited just once. Why has this stuck so firmly in your memory even though you made absolutely no attempt to memorize it? Visual memories stick. This makes sense based on our evolution. When we were more primitive animals, survival was based on our ability to travel away from the home, find food, and successfully make it back to shelter. The ability to memorize landscapes and travel paths made the difference between life and death. So our brains evolved to develop the natural ability to memorize locations and visual images. What our brains are naturally terrible at doing is memorizing lists of information, numbers, and tons of facts. This was not necessary for survival as we evolved. But this is exactly what we ask our brains to do throughout our education.

The trick to memorizing is to combine our visual memories with the long lists of information we have to remember. Here is a demonstration. For this to work, you must make an attempt to follow along and try it yourself. We will start by trying to memorize another list of twenty random words.

First picture the home you are most familiar with. It could be the one you are currently living in or perhaps your childhood home. Now I want you to start outside your front door. Imagine standing there, and next to you is a *newspaper*. Think hard about the visual image with your eyes closed until it truly appears in your head. Make it as memorable as possible by picturing a huge newspaper blocking your path or perhaps falling onto you. The crazier the image, the better. This will be the place where you remember the word *newspaper*. Now walk into the front door, and just as you walk in, you see a *camel*. Visualize it standing there, perhaps doing something crazy like spitting at you. Close your eyes and picture the camel in your house. What does it look like? Next walk into the adjoining room and picture *Abraham Lincoln*. Close your eyes, and picture him! What is he doing? Is he sitting there or running around? Continue your walk through your house in an orderly way, and in every new place you walk, put another one of the words listed on the next page. But remember to picture it firmly before you move onto the next word and next location in your home. The crazier you can make these images, the better. Try to incorporate as many of your senses into the memory. How does the object feel? Does it smell bad? Above all, use your imagination!

Fire hydrant	Soccer ball
Concrete	Eagle
Laptop	Orange
Oatmeal	Screwdriver
Broken collar bone	Pen
Blanket	Oil
Diamonds	Surfboard
Hail	Justice
Strep throat	Street
Scissors	Barrel

Done? Now walk back through your house, and try to list off each word as you walk through. How many did you recall? If you did this right, you should easily be able to recall almost all of the words, if not all of them. This is how rote memorization can be transformed into a much easier system.

You may have found it difficult to memorize some words more than others. For example, the word "justice" has no distinct visual that comes up. So we have to make one up. You may have pictured a courtroom or a supreme court justice. The bottom line is that you should let your imagination run free. The more senses you can incorporate apart from just visual (such as feeling the orange or imagining how it smells) will make it that much easier to recall. Make the images stand out by distorting them or giving them actions. Our brains are also very good at memorizing when it involves erotic images, again likely because sex is important for survival of a species from an evolution standpoint. The bottom line is to make it stick in your head. Once you practice, you will find more effective ways to make images memorable.

How much more efficient is this system than simple repetition? Try this test. Tomorrow try to recall words from both of the lists. Don't look back now! See how many you still remember. Be sure to walk through your house again when you try to recall the second list.

"But wait," you say. "I don't have to memorize lists of objects. I have to memorize much more difficult information that I can't easily visualize."

Let's say you have an anatomy test and need to remember the layers of the epidermis. Words in medicine are not so straightforward as memorizing lists of common words. Although memorization of medical terminology does not come as easily, with a little bit of imagination you can still apply the same concepts. For example the layers of the epidermis are the following:

Stratum corneum

Stratum lucidum

Stratum granulosum

Stratum spinosum

Stratum basale

Picture a room in your house with a catwalk, and you are *strutting* your stuff as you walk along it. This will help you remember that each of these words will begin with the word "stratum." As you are strutting down, the object you run into first is a huge eyeball. Picture the white *cornea* as you pick up the eyeball. Or alternatively think of a huge ear of *corn*. Either way you've just remembered the first layer, stratum corneum. You keep walking down the catwalk, and next you run into *Lucy* from the show *I Love Lucy*. This helps you remember the next layer is stratum lucidum. She asks you why you're carrying a big eyeball. But you don't have time to talk. You have to keep strutting past her, and as you walk, you run into your grandma. She owes Lucy some money. You tell her, *"Gran, you owe some."* And this helps you remember stratum granulosum. She pinches your cheeks, and you keep on strutting. You step over a book that is well balanced on its *spine*, and you have now remembered stratum spinosum. Finally at the end, you see a home plate. You slide and touch the *base*. Just like that, you've finished your walk down the catwalk, and you have also remembered the last layer of the epidermis, the stratum basale. Now, take a visual walk down the catwalk and see if you remember each layer.

Walk through it again tomorrow and maybe in a week, and you may find that you can remember the layers of the epidermis for the rest of your life. That's the power of visual memory.

In this example I've also shown you another trick, which is to create a story. You might not have enough unique spots in your house to put all of the various tidbits of information. But in each location, you could potentially place multiple pieces of information by creating a story. This catwalk I just mentioned can easily be shoved into a small corner of your room where it will stay and help you remember five distinct names.

You can use this as a fun party trick as well. Walk through your house and identify fifty unique spaces you will use. This is called creating a memory palace. Make sure you know exactly where each space is, and remember the way you will walk through the house to remember all fifty spaces in the same order. Now have someone slowly call off fifty random words. After each word take some time to ensure you have visualized it well, then ask for the next word. Once all fifty spaces are filled, walk back through your memory palace and amaze your friends with how great your memory is. Anyone can do it, thanks to evolution!

Chapter 26

The Anatomy Lab

The popular media depicts the anatomy lab as a rite of passage for medical students. Dissecting human cadavers is seen as the ultimate test to determine if your nerves and stomach are strong enough to be a doctor. I remember being nervous about starting this course. Would I be able to handle the smell or make it through dissections without getting nauseated? It wasn't until the lab began that I realized how wrong many of my preconceived notions were. It is for that reason that I've dedicated this chapter to explaining the real story behind the anatomy lab and providing some relief to the anxiety.

First and foremost the lab is not a rite of passage. It is similar to every other class. It is an instructional course dedicated to furthering your medical knowledge. Although some students will always have difficulty dealing with the sights and smells of the lab, your instructors and fellow students should help you get through the experience, not ostracize you because you are "weak."

The lab will serve as a supplement to your gross anatomy course. It will make tangible all of the various muscles, organs, nerves, and bones you will learn about in your textbook. Use this time to truly learn how this incredible machine called the human body is built. After all you will be the mechanic for the rest of your career.

Although it will be tempting to hide your nervousness about human dissection through jokes and humor, remember the sacrifice that was made to give you this opportunity. These individuals decided to donate their bodies for your education. Show that you appreciate this sacrifice by respecting the process of dissecting the body, and use the opportunity to learn.

For those who have read this chapter and still worry about the difficulty in handling the smell of preservatives and sights in the lab, here are some tricks to help:

1. For those who are particularly sensitive to smells, try breathing through your mouth to limit any unpleasant odors from reaching your smell receptors. Some labs also have special masks that can be worn to help limit the smell. Sprinkling some perfume or cologne on the inside of the mask may also help. Some advocate chewing cinnamon gum, but I never tried this, so I can't comment on its effectiveness. If all else fails, one of my instructors recommended getting close to the cadaver at the beginning of the lab and taking some deep breaths to fully saturate

your smell receptors, thereby desensitizing you to the smell.

2. For those who feel queasy at the site of blood and a deceased body, try to desensitize by watching videos of dissections on YouTube. Also once the lab starts, force yourself to jump in and get involved. Sometimes the fear of being uneasy makes us even more uneasy. Once we jump in, the fear goes away.

3. Think about the science. For each part you dissect, try to think back to your coursework, and use the opportunity to learn about each of the body parts. The visual will help cement your knowledge. By approaching it academically, sometimes the uneasiness is lessened.

Overall the anatomy lab is an incredible experience. Take the opportunity to truly appreciate the complex and dynamic human body. Respect the sacrifice made by the cadavers and their families. And remember you will never have this opportunity again. Take full advantage of it!

Chapter 27
Overview of the Rotations

The transition into medical school rotations is perhaps the most challenging part of medical school. Students go from the warm, comfortable lecture room they've called home over the last twenty years to suddenly being thrown into a brand-new learning environment. This environment is filled with anxiety, uncertainty, and a constant sense of being scrutinized and graded. However, with the proper attitude and preparation, medical school rotations can be a very rewarding, satisfying, and educational experience. During these rotations students truly start to learn how to be doctors.

Each rotation will likely consist of both an inpatient and outpatient component. The inpatient component deals with the patients who are admitted to the hospital for acute health issues. The outpatient component consists of clinics in which the patient comes to the doctor for a specific health concern or regular checkup, the doctor makes recommendations, and then the patient goes home.

As far as the structure of the inpatient component, almost all rotations have a very similar organization. The team is headed by one doctor who is in charge of care.

This doctor is called the attending. The attending doctor is at the top of the medical totem pole. Next on the totem pole is the resident. Residency training programs can last anywhere from three to eight or more years, depending on the specialty. Once residents complete residency training, they will become attendings. Next is the intern. This title is given to a resident who is in the first year of residency. The intern is fresh out of medical school and oftentimes is still learning the ropes. Most of the work is done by the intern and resident. The attending is the final authority in charge of the patient's care. The attending's job is to ensure that the team is making the appropriate medical decisions.

A typical day will start with the intern and resident coming in very early. They will first talk with the team that was covering the patients overnight to get "sign-out." During this time the overnight team will update the daytime team on any new concerns or issues that have arisen and briefly discuss each patient to transition their care. Next the resident and intern will gather all the data that are necessary to make medical decisions. This includes getting any new lab results or radiology results, gathering vital signs, talking to the nursing staff, and examining the patients. This is known as "prerounding." Once the patient is examined and all of the data are gathered, the team will then meet with the attending. They may sit down in a conference room and discuss each patient on the list, or they may walk around to every patient's room and discuss each case. This is known as "rounding." The team will take all the information that has been gathered so far and decide on a plan of action for that day. Rounding will usually take a few hours in the morning, but if all goes well, it should be completed prior to noon that day. Residents and interns will use whatever time they have left in the day to enter new orders, admit new patients, discharge patients who are ready to go home, update patients on plans, and complete medical notes. Each patient needs a note in the medical record that details the patient's progress and overall plan of care.

So where do medical students fit into this equation? Medical students are an additional part of the medical teams. The main job of the medical student is to practice how eventually to assume the role of an intern. This process is done by going through the same process that the intern goes through. Medical students will be assigned certain patients who they will examine and collect data on during prerounding, and they will present the case to the attending during formal rounds. However, doctors do realize that medical students are still learning. Therefore you never have the last say when it comes to medical decisions, and you should be provided with adequate amounts of supervision to ensure patients get appropriate care. Most of the time, residents and interns will work in parallel with medical students and will also examine patients and collect information even though a medical student is assigned to that same patient. There should always be supervision of care.

Perhaps the most challenging and anxiety-provoking time during rotations is rounding with the entire team. A good portion of your grade is based on how well you do during this time. Medical students will be in charge of presenting each of their patients during morning rounds. For new patients this consists of going through the entire medical history. For follow-up patients, it consists of specifically discussing overnight events, the current examination, new labs/studies, and care for that day. Presenting patients can be nerve-racking because all eyes are on you during the presentation. It is also the time in which you may be asked medical questions to test your knowledge. This process is commonly referred to as pimping. We will talk more about presenting patients and pimping later in this book.

Most medical schools begin core rotations during the third year. These rotations typically consist of internal medicine, surgery, obstetrics and gynecology, family medicine, psychiatry, neurology, and pediatrics. Each of these rotations comes with its separate sets of challenges and obstacles. Let's review some general tips for getting the best grade on rotations. Then we will review each rotation and discuss strategies on how to survive and thrive!

Chapter 28

Keys to Getting Honors

It's everyone's goal to get a grade of honors during each rotation. A grade of honors looks very good on a transcript and increases the chances of getting the residency of your choice. Here is a quick summary of the main tips that apply to all rotations.

1. Be on time. As a medical student, you should never delay the team in any way. It is critical for you to show up early for rounds. I have never seen a medical student show up persistently late, and I guarantee it's a surefire way of getting a low grade.

2. Be enthusiastic. No matter what rotation you are in, you should be an enthusiastic member of the team and take interest in your patients. Residents are often tired and grumpy. They do not want to be around other tired and grumpy people. Don't overdo it either. I've seen students go overboard. Fake enthusiasm is annoying.

3. Work as a team. All of medicine requires teamwork. Getting along with other members of the team is important, including fellow medical students, nursing staff, front desk staff, janitors, and anybody else who works in the hospital. Residents will take notice of how you interact

with others. Part of your grade will undoubtedly be your professional demeanor. So do not be overly competitive, and never do anything to undercut a fellow student.

4. Help the team. If tasks need to be done, even if they sound trivial, it is important to pitch in. Not everything in medicine is as dramatic as you see on TV shows. Sometimes getting medical records from another hospital is as exciting as it gets for a student, and that's okay. Anything you do to help the team is helping the patient.

5. Have clear and crisp presentations. This is perhaps one of the most important things you can do. For a new patient presentation, you should have practiced it a few times before rounds. Think of these presentations as a performance. You should practice your performance so you do the best possible job. A confident, clear, yet succinct presentation is key to obtaining honors on any rotation.

6. Stay organized and look professional. Students are expected to come to work in professional attire. You should be well groomed. You shouldn't be stumbling around with tons of papers; have a very organized way of collecting all of your materials. Don't be sloppy.

7. Know your patients well. As a student, you are expected to know your patients better than anyone else simply

because you have more time to get to know them. Spend time talking to the families and reviewing patients' charts.

8. Take ownership. If you are covering a patient, that is your patient! You should feel the responsibility to make sure everything gets done for this patient.

9. Take initiative. Don't expect the resident to always give you a list of tasks. Listen during rounds, and be proactive about finding work to do. Try to make the resident's workday more efficient by getting things done.

Chapter 29

Advice for Specific Rotations

Every rotation during medical school comes with its own set of challenges. Let's discuss the best approach to each of these unique experiences.

Internal Medicine

Internal medicine is perhaps one of the most challenging rotations during the third year. Any adult medical problem that does not fit neatly within another subspecialty category usually ends up on the internal medicine service. This means internal medicine physicians see a wide variety of medical problems and pathologic processes. And although learning all of internal medicine during a medical student rotation is impossible, this will be the rotation where you will probably learn the most during your third year.

Most internal medicine residents are very hardworking and intelligent. A strong emphasis is on evidence-based medicine. This means that people rely on data from research studies to determine which medications and treatments work best for various diseases. One key to doing well on internal medicine is knowing the disease process as well as knowing some of the recent literature on that particular disease. One very good resource is UpToDate.com, to which certain hospitals have a subscription. On this website you will find reviews of various diseases as well as discussions on recent research studies that pertain to the topic. This website can be helpful for other rotations as well, but it is probably the most useful during internal medicine.

Given the strong emphasis on evidence-based medicine, if you do find recent articles in respected journals that pertain to your patient's disease, most residents and attendings will be impressed if you e-mail the team this article or talk briefly about it during your patient presentations. But every team is different, and every resident is different. Try to get a feel for whether this will be a welcome addition or a time-consuming nuisance for the residents.

Recommended Reading: *First Aid for the Medicine Clerkship* by Matthew Kaufman.

Surgery

The surgery rotation can be challenging. Not only are there long hours, but the stereotype is that most surgery residents and attendings are abrasive and hard to work with. Surgery as a field requires a certain type of attitude. Most surgeons tend to be very focused and goal-oriented and can be very direct with their language. They also tend to be very overworked, which can contribute to fatigue and irritability. This situation can make for a challenging work environment for the medical student. But like all rotations, a bit of your experience depends simply on the people with whom you are paired. There are plenty of friendly surgery residents.

The key to doing well on the surgery rotation is developing a surgeon-like mentality. This means working hard and being efficient. Most surgery residents appreciate a very succinct presentation during rounds. They respect healthy confidence and appreciate medical students who can help out with tasks that need to be done.

This tends to be one of the more thrilling rotations because students get to watch surgeries and often participate as well. Students are taught the appropriate way to sterilize themselves to participate in a surgery. Paying attention to the sterilization technique is crucial because this will prevent you from contaminating a patient during surgery. Breaking the sterile field during a surgery is a very quick way to get a bad grade.

Students are often asked to help with small tasks during the surgery, such as cutting or tying sutures and holding back flaps of skin while the surgery proceeds. I found it helpful to learn a bit about each surgical procedure prior to going into the operating room. A great reference book to quickly review surgical procedures is *Surgical Recall*. I was able to answer many questions that the surgeon asked during surgery because I reviewed the case just prior.

Recommended reading: *Surgical Recall* by Lorne Blackbourne.

Obstetrics and Gynecology

One of the most amazing experiences as a medical student is delivering your first baby. This is where it becomes clear that you are well on your way to becoming a doctor. Although the OBGYN rotation can be challenging due to long hours, it is also a specialty that has many cases that become routine, and therefore it gives you the chance to become comfortable treating many of the common conditions. Residents in OBGYN may have a reputation of being mean and abrasive, but in my experience I found this to be untrue.

Like any rotation in medical school, the key to doing well in the OBGYN rotation is showing enthusiasm and interest in the field. Even if you know that you don't want to go into OBGYN, making an active effort to learn and stay engaged during your rotation is important. This may also be the first time you learn the proper techniques for scrubbing into surgery. The keys to getting honors on the OBGYN rotation are to be an active part of the team and seek out opportunities to participate in procedures whenever possible.

Recommended reading: *Obstetrics and Gynecology* by Charles Beckmann, et al.

Family Medicine

The family medicine rotation tends to be more relaxed than most other rotations. This is due to a combination of limited work hours because family medicine is mostly an outpatient experience, as well as faculty that are usually very personable and approachable. The cases vary quite widely, but you will develop comfort with some of the more common reasons for visits to a family medicine doctor, including management of upper respiratory infections, diabetes, hypertension, and high cholesterol. The family medicine rotation is a good time to practice physical exams because patients do not tend to be acutely ill and therefore are more cooperative with medical students.

The keys to doing well include finding ways to make clinic more efficient for the provider. Because the day can be busy with many appointments, find a role you can play to help your attending. This could include writing notes, ordering/checking labs, or making patient phone calls. Try to get involved as much as possible in the clinic. You will learn more this way.

Recommended Reading: *Case Files Family Medicine* by Eugene Toy.

Pediatrics

Often considered the most lighthearted of medical school rotations, pediatrics can also be challenging. Dealing with sick children is not easy. However, the rotation overall tends to be an enjoyable one for students. The residents and attendings in pediatrics tend to be friendlier than in other specialties.

The key to getting honors is to be friendly and approachable. This is not the time to bring out the surgery mentality. Interact with patients and families, and spend time discussing the plans of care. Try to keep the medical team informed of the family's concerns. This is one rotation with many moving parts, given the fact that the patient is not the primary decision maker and parents are very particular about their children's care, as they should be.

Physical examinations on children can be challenging depending on the child's age. Try to approach the child playfully at first, then focus on the examination. The best examinations are a combination of playing and examining, such as asking the child to hold your stethoscope and place it on the heart themselves.

Recommended reading: *Blueprints in Pediatrics* by Bradley Marino and Katie Fine.

Psychiatry

At first the psychiatry rotation can be a bit disconcerting. We are accustomed to interacting with people in a predictable way. During this rotation people's behavior may not always be predictable, which leads to discomfort. Heeding precautions from residents and attendings regarding certain patients during the psychiatry rotation is important. You need to know when to call for help should you get into a situation that makes you uncomfortable. If you are interviewing a mentally unstable individual, the patient should not be between you and the door. But remember that most patients in psychiatry have no intention of hurting others. As the psychiatry rotation continues, you will find that the majority of cases involve regular people in difficult situations.

The psychiatry rotation can be a very eye-opening rotation. You often come face-to-face with some of the most difficult social situations. Although many cases may be upsetting or disheartening, it is also a rotation in which many patients improve over time.

Similar to the rotation in OBGYN, the material covered during psychiatry is not excessively extensive. Wrapping your head around the main disorders and becoming very familiar with treatment strategies is possible. Also similar to OBGYN, many students come into the rotation knowing for certain that they do not intend to go into this specialty. However, once again, the key to doing well is to show interest and take this opportunity to learn about disorders that you will likely encounter again in the future.

The other key to doing well is to take a very thorough history. The history in psychiatry is everything. Paying particular attention to the social history is vital. Getting comfortable asking the difficult questions is also important during this rotation, such as thoughts of suicide or homicide, history of sexual abuse, and drug use.

Recommended Reading: *First Aid for the Psychiatry Clerkship* by Latha Ganti.

Neurology

During the neurology rotation, students will see a variety of pathologies. Residents and attendings in neurology have a reputation of being somewhat quirky individuals. At their core most neurologists are very intellectual people and are the epitome of academicians. The key to doing well on this rotation is becoming familiar with the neurologic examination and learning to present a thorough yet succinct physical exam. At the end of your presentations, always try to localize where the problem is occurring. The nervous system extends all the way from the brain to the peripheral nerves and muscles. Is there a problem in the brain? If so, which part of the brain? Do you feel the problem is in the spine, and if so, what parts of the neurologic exam point toward a spinal cord lesion? Performing a thorough neurologic exam and using this to help pinpoint the location of the disease process will gain you big points during this rotation. It is always nice to run your thoughts by the resident to ensure they agree prior to presenting it during rounds.

The presentation of the neurologic exam should follow the same pattern every time. The main categories in the neurologic examination include mental status, cranial nerves, motor exam, sensory exam, reflexes, coordination, and gait. They should be presented in this order unless specified differently by a resident. Learn how to test all of the components in each category, and practice repeatedly. Try practicing the exam on normal individuals. Perform the neurologic exam on friends and family. Only after establishing a good sense of "normal" will you then be able to identify pathology.

Please note that for every other rotation, the neurologic exam will be more succinct. Often times simply saying, "no focal deficits" will suffice for this exam. But for the neurology rotation, details are important. Here is an example of how to present a normal neurologic exam during the neurology rotation. Don't worry if you do not recognize all of the terminology. This should be taught to you prior to the rotation.

Mental Status: The patient was awake, alert, and oriented to person, place, and time. Her language was normal, and she was able to name objects.

Cranial Nerves: Pupils were equally round and reactive to light, extra-ocular movements were intact, V1 through V3 sensation was normal, face was symmetric to smile, hearing was intact to finger rub bilaterally, palate elevated equally, sternocleidomastoid and trapezius strength were 5 out of 5, and tongue protrusion was midline.

Motor: The patient had 5 out of 5 strength in upper and lower extremities. Normal muscle bulk and tone.

Sensory: The patient had normal sensation to light touch, pinprick, temperature, vibration, and proprioception in upper and lower extremities.

Reflexes: 2+ reflexes in upper and lower extremities. Toes were down-going on Babinski testing.

Coordination: Finger-to-nose was normal. Heel-to-shin was normal.

Gait: The patient had a normal gait. She could walk in tandem, on heels and toes. Romberg testing was negative.

Recommended reading: *Clinical Neuroanatomy Made Ridiculously Simple* by Stephen Goldberg.

Chapter 30

Pre-Rounding Strategies

As we discussed before, the key to obtaining a high grade during rotations is a great presentation during rounds. A great presentation starts with a thorough knowledge of the patient's history, exam, and relevant workup. Prerounding is the process in which you collect information about your patient and examine them prior to official rounds with the attending and the entire team. The most important way to approach prerounding is that of a steady jog, not a frantic sprint to collect all the data.

Create a strategy for collecting data in the most efficient and thorough way possible. For me this process started by listening to sign-out from the overnight on-call team. The overnight team provides very pertinent information about what happened the night before and will help determine which patients may need extra attention and time during prerounding. Without knowing what happened to the patient overnight, it is very hard to get a sense of which direction the patient is going. If you were not able to hear sign-out from the on-call team, try to touch base with the intern who is covering the patient to get a quick rundown. Be sure that this does not interfere with the intern's prerounding or you run the risk of making him or her irritated. Another way to get information about overnight events is to talk to the nurse taking care of the patient. I found this to be the best way to find out about overnight events if I couldn't hear it directly from the overnight team. After all, during my first year of rotations, I wouldn't often get to the hospital early enough to hear sign-out directly from the on-call team, so nurses were my main source of information. Next I would typically sit down at the computer and gather lab results, radiology results, and any other testing that was new from the day prior. Finally I would examine each patient and collect his/her vital signs. This includes temperature, blood pressure, respiratory rate, heart rate, and oxygen saturation. These should already be documented by nurses.

If your hospital lab draw is late in the morning, the results might not be back if you are prerounding very early. In this case you may want to examine each patient prior to collecting lab data.

If you're using an electronic medical record system, there are often ways to set up alerts so you are informed of every new lab that has come back for your patients. Sit down with residents, and learn the shortcuts early in your rotation. It will make prerounding much more efficient.

Once you've examined each patient, collected vital signs, reviewed the laboratory data, and spoken with the overnight nurse, sitting down and thinking about your plans for the patient prior to formal rounds is helpful. If you have a helpful intern and resident, they will often discuss the plan with you prior to formal rounds so you have some idea of what to say before presenting in front of the attending. Doing this will make you much more confident in your presentation.

When covering multiple patients, I found it very helpful to have a rounding sheet. Such a sheet makes it easy for you to keep track of all of the data for multiple patients. I have put the rounding sheet I used online for you to download and print. You can modify this rounding sheet in the way that suits your needs. You can find the rounding sheet at http://goo.gl/M7ardW.

Chapter 31

Presenting Your Patients

During formal rounds, you will be expected to present your patients to the entire team. Every medical student is nervous during this time. It would be highly unusual if you were not. Rest assured that as the years go by, confidence slowly replaces this nervousness. But that takes time. I was well into my intern year before my heart stopped racing before every patient presentation.

I found that practicing my presentations made it much easier for me to present and made me more confident. You need to be succinct, yet thorough. As a resident and attending, I was always impressed when a medical student could get through a presentation without too many pauses and without frequently saying, *um* and *uh*. Formal rounds should not be the first time in which you read through your presentation. You should have already thought about what you were going to say and made sure that your presentation makes sense. This will be the time in which most of your grade is decided; you must put your best foot forward.

In the very beginning of the rotation, try to sit down with the resident to get a better understanding of your expectations during rounds. Ask the residents up front which parts of the presentation they would like for you to present, how they would like to hear it, and whether they would like to hear details about vital signs and lab results. Some residents are comfortable with you saying that the vital signs are normal and that there were no abnormal lab results. Some residents want you to list out every vital sign and lab result. There is no right or wrong way. The right way is essentially what will work best for your particular team and provides the best care for patients.

As far as the format of the presentation, please see chapter 33 on writing notes; your presentation should essentially follow the same structure.

Chapter 32

How to Handle Pimping

As you may know, the term pimping describes the process in which residents and attendings will ask you various medical questions to test your knowledge. Similar to the presentation, this is also a time that produces a great deal of anxiety for the medical student. After all, your knowledge is being tested, often in front of the entire medical team. Students may feel that their grades depend on how they answer these questions.

The first thing to realize as a student is that you're not expected to know everything. As a medical student I often put undue pressure on myself to know all of the answers to questions and would feel stupid if I didn't have the right answer. Not until residency did I realize that no one expects medical students to have the answers. Even interns are not expected to know many answers because they are still early in the learning phase. In fact everyone is still learning, even the attendings. Although medical students do know a great deal of information, you should not feel embarrassed if you are unable to answer a question during rounds. It is also important to develop a comfort saying the words, "I don't know." It's okay not to know every answer. If you already had all of the answers, you would not be paying medical school tuition to learn. I also feel that a confident "I don't know" sometimes comes across better than nervously searching for the answer even if you eventually come up with the right answer. Students should also understand that when residents and attendings ask questions, it is not typically used to determine how smart you are as a student. Instead it is typically used by doctors to find holes in your medical knowledge so they can teach. Don't feel as though you are constantly being tested. (Check out chapter 5 of my book *Everything I Learned in Medical School* to read about my medical student experience with pimping.)

Of course it is nice to answer questions correctly when being pimped. Learning about the disease process for your patients is vital. Go home and learn about the pathophysiology, typical clinical presentations for the disease, and rationale behind treatment approaches. Most questions during rounds will come from your patient's case.

An etiquette also comes along with pimping. Although some may show off knowledge by answering questions addressed to other students, it is more prudent to remain a team player and show solidarity with your classmates. Do not display your medical knowledge at the expense of others. Showing that you can be a part of the team will be reflected in your grade. Of course if they ask you the question directly after your classmate could not figure out the answer, you do not have to feign ignorance. But answer in a way that makes you look sympathetic to your classmate. So you shouldn't say, "It's obviously sarcoid." You would instead say something to the effect of, "I believe this could be sarcoid."

Chapter 33

Writing a Good Note

Proper documentation is vital in medicine. It is how patient care is communicated between providers for continuity of care. Good notes are also helpful for your own reference during future encounters with the same patient. And if that's not reason enough, remember that we live in an increasingly litigious society. So documenting everything you do is important. All patients should have a daily progress note while in the hospital. Each outpatient encounter should have a clinic note that documents the details of that visit.

When you are seeing the patient for the first time, whether it is an inpatient or outpatient, the structure of the note is very similar. It is called a History and Physical (H&P). The following is the main format:

1. Chief complaint (CC): This is the complaint that the patient presents with. Oftentimes the attending may request that the chief complaint be in the patient's own words. Therefore the chief complaint should not be "evaluate for heart attack." Instead it should be "pain in my chest." Chief complaints should only be a few words and at most one sentence.

2. History of present illness (HPI): This section should essentially be a story that presents a history of the current chief complaint. It usually starts off with one line that states the age and sex of the patient with a summary of the pertinent medical problems. For example, the history of present illness for somebody presenting with chest pain may start off with, "The patient is a fifty-five-year-old male with a history of one prior heart attack who presents with two hours of chest pain." In that one sentence, I managed to adequately describe the patient's pertinent background and reason for evaluation, thereby laying the groundwork for the rest of the HPI and presentation. Attendings like to have this foundation so they know what bits of information they will need to garner from your presentation. The rest of the HPI should present what led up to this chest pain and provide a description of the symptoms themselves. Therefore the remainder of the HPI may go as follows: "The patient was in his usual state of health until this afternoon when he was shoveling snow in his driveway. After fifteen minutes of shoveling snow, the patient reports he began experiencing chest pain. He describes the pain as a crushing sensation incorporating the left side of his chest. He describes the pain as nine out of ten in intensity. The pain radiated to his left arm. The pain was associated with shortness of breath as well as sweating. The pain persisted despite resting for fifteen minutes, and therefore an ambulance was called and brought him to the emergency room."

3. Past medical history (PMH): After the HPI, present the patient's full past medical history. Listing the pertinent medical conditions first is important. For the patient coming in with chest pain, you would talk about his cardiac history. For your notes, be as thorough as possible with the PMH. However, during your presentations, the resident and attendings might not want every detail of the patient's PMH (e.g., the ingrown toenail from ten years ago) and only expect to hear about the pertinent parts.

4. Medications: This is where you'll list all of the patient's home medications. A thorough note will also have the doses of each medication and the route through which it is administered (by mouth, inhaled, etc.).

5. Allergies: Allergies to medications should be listed in this section, as well as the nature of the reaction (rash, anaphylaxis, etc.). Many people will report something as an allergy because they experienced an adverse reaction, such as constipation. This is not considered a true allergy, so ask about the reaction to determine if there is evidence of an allergic response (such as rash, swelling, hives, vomiting, difficulty breathing, etc.). If there are no allergies, write "NKDA," which stands for "No known drug allergies."

6. Family history: You should list the pertinent diseases that run in the family in this section. For a patient presenting with a cardiac problem, you will need to discuss family history of cardiac disease, hypertension, diabetes, and other factors that play a role in causing heart problems. Start by asking patients about the relevant problems, and then open it up and ask if anything else runs in the family.

7. Social history: For adults the social history typically consists of information on alcohol use, smoking, and sexual history. It may also be important to describe the living situation and discuss any barriers, such as financial constraints, that could affect future care and access to medications.

8. Review of systems (ROS): Exactly as it sounds, this section is a review of the various organ systems to see if the patient has any other symptoms that aren't necessarily brought up in the HPI. There are fourteen categories recognized within the review of systems. These categories are constitutional symptoms, eyes, ear/nose/throat (ENT), cardiovascular, respiratory, gastrointestinal, genital/urinary, musculoskeletal, integumentary/breast, neurological, psychiatric, endocrine, hematologic/lymph, and allergic/immunologic. Here is a list of the typical symptoms that are relevant for each category:

A. Constitutional: fatigue, weight change, fever, chills

B. Eyes: visual loss, double vision, blurred vision

C. ENT: hearing loss, ear pain, congestion, runny nose

D. Cardiovascular: chest pain, palpitations, chest discomfort, edema

E. Respiratory: shortness of breath, cough, wheezing

F. Gastrointestinal: nausea, vomiting, diarrhea, heartburn, abdominal pain

G. Genital/urinary: Burning on urination, urgency, loss of bladder/bowel control

H. Musculoskeletal: muscle pain, back pain, cramps, joint pain, stiffness

I. Integumentary/breast: breast pain, soreness, lumps

J. Neurological: headache, weakness, dizziness, numbness

K. Psychiatric: depression, anxiety

L. Endocrine: sweating, cold or heat intolerance

M. Hematologic/lymphatic: anemia, bleeding, bruising, enlarged lymph nodes

N. Allergic/immunologic: asthma, hives, eczema, swelling

Will you ask a patient about every single symptom? Probably not depending on the time constraints. Simply ask if anything else is bothering the person currently, with a particular emphasis on systems that are pertinent to the chief complaint. For example, with a heart attack patients often get nauseated. This would be a relevant point in the ROS.

9. Physical exam (PE): The physical exam should start with a summary of the vital signs (temperature, heart rate, blood pressure, respiratory rate). Next is typically a general examination, which is an overall impression of how the patient looks. This is followed by cardiovascular, respiratory, and the abdominal exam. These parts are considered the core of any physical examination. From there you can examine other areas that you feel are pertinent to the patient's case.

10. Assessment: Start the assessment with a one-line summary of the patient's presentation. Then discuss the differential diagnosis (which is a list of the various things that could be causing the patient's problem) and your thought process behind the differential diagnosis. Decide what you believe to be the most likely cause of the patient's chief complaint.

11. Plan: This is a detailed list of what you intend to do with the patient, such as further workup or initiation of treatment. It is based on your assessment of what is causing the patient's health problems.

The following is an example of a full H&P for a patient being admitted to the hospital. Remember that your written note and presentation should follow the same format. All new patients should have an H&P regardless of whether they are being seen in the clinic or in the hospital.

Chief complaint: "I keep passing out."

History of present illness: The patient is a sixteen-year-old male who is being evaluated for recurrent episodes of losing consciousness. The patient reports that he was otherwise healthy until approximately five months ago when he had his first episode of losing consciousness. He was otherwise feeling well at that time without any illness. He stayed up late the night prior playing video games. In the morning when he woke up, he remembers coming down to the kitchen but does not recall feeling poorly. The next thing he remembers is waking up in the ambulance. The mother reports that after he walked into the kitchen, he suddenly developed a blank stare, slumped to the ground, and then began shaking all of his extremities. She reports that his eyes were open and rolled back. The shaking lasted for two minutes and then stopped on its own. After the shaking stopped, the patient was very tired and sleepy but able to respond to simple questions. He did not have any urinary incontinence or tongue biting. He was evaluated in the emergency department at that time with a CT scan of his brain and was sent home after he returned back to baseline. He experienced a second similar episode today, which is again described as suddenly losing consciousness. Bystanders witnessed the event and describe all of his extremities shaking with eyes rolled back. This episode lasted thirty minutes, and the shaking did not stop until EMS arrived and administered intramuscular midazolam. After one hour, he awoke and has been able to answer questions. He denies fever, drug use, or any other triggers. He is being admitted for further evaluation.

Past medical history: Mild asthma, seasonal allergies.

Medications: Albuterol as needed, fluticasone nasal spray daily.

Allergies: Penicillin causes a rash.

Family history: There is no family history of seizures. There is a cousin with autism. No other neurologic problems run in the family. Mother has a history of hypertension and anxiety. Father has a history of coronary artery disease.

Social history: He lives at home with his parents and younger brother. He is in the tenth grade. He makes As and Bs. He denies alcohol or drug abuse. He is not sexually active.

Review of systems: (Note: when presenting the history during rounds, only mention the pertinent items.) Constitutional: No fevers, no weight loss. Eyes: No vision changes. ENT: Intermittent runny nose from his allergies. Cardiovascular: No chest pain or shortness of breath. Respiratory: Intermittent cough at nighttime. Gastrointestinal: No constipation or diarrhea. Genital/urinary: No urgency. Musculoskeletal: No muscle pain or stiffness. Neurological: As per HPI. Psychiatric: No history of depression or anxiety. Endocrine: No heat or cold intolerance. Hematologic/lymphatic: No bruising. Allergic/Immunologic: No hives.

Assessment: This is a sixteen-year-old presenting with his second episode of loss of consciousness with full-body shaking. The description of the event does sound consistent with a seizure. Other possibilities include syncope (from dehydration, cardiac arrhythmia, or vasovagal syncope), as well as pseudoseizures.

Plan: Admit patient to the hospital for observation given the length of the event. Obtain an EEG to evaluate for abnormal discharges while he is here. Obtain an MRI to ensure there are no problems with the structure of his brain. Finally, start him on seizure medications because this most likely represents two unprovoked seizures. I will plan to start him on Levetiracetam five hundred milligrams twice a day. The family will need education about seizure first aid. He should have a prescription for rectal valium in case of a prolonged seizure.

If the patient has already had pertinent lab work or radiology images done during this hospitalization, it is typical to list those after the physical exam section.

If you think of every new patient in the above format, you will not miss anything important. Over time you'll learn the pertinent positives and negatives for various presenting problems and efficiently perform the entire history and physical. Sometimes patients can get off topic and continue to elaborate without adding substantial information to their medical issues. This is where the art of medicine comes into play. You'll soon learn how to redirect patients in a polite and professional manner, thereby allowing them to get back on topic.

If the patient is in the hospital, they will have a progress note each day after the day of admission. Progress notes are not as detailed as the H&P and usually follow the "SOAP" format (which stands for subjective, objective, assessment, and plan). The following is an example of a progress note for the above patient:

Subjective: 16yo male admitted for second unprovoked seizure. Well overnight and at his baseline. No further seizure activity. He reports some muscle soreness, but otherwise well this morning.

Objective: Vitals: T-98.4, RR-12, BP-107/73, HR-80.

Labs/Work-up: EEG-normal, MRI: no lesions, normal brain.

Medications: Levetiracetam 500mg BID

Assessment: 16yo male admitted after second unprovoked seizure. His workup thus far is normal, however children with epilepsy can have normal MRI and EEG.

Plan: 1. Continue Levetiracetam 500mg twice a day.

2. Complete seizure first aid education for patient and family.

3. Discharge home today with outpatient follow-up in pediatric neurology clinic in two weeks.

Although a SOAP note is typical for following a patient in the hospital, follow-up notes for patients seen in clinics vary depending on the specialty. But the general content to follow-up notes includes a reason for the visit, notable changes since the last visit, updated medical history, medications, physical exam, and an assessment/plan at the end.

Chapter 34

Calling for a Consult

During your inpatient rotation, the team may require the evaluation of a patient by a subspecialty team. For example while on internal medicine, you may have a patient with a severe pneumonia for whom you would like the opinion of the infectious disease specialists. Calling a subspecialist to get his/her opinion on a case is known as calling a consult. Residents often appreciate if the medical student can call consults for his or her patients. However, calling a consult can be nerve-racking. Oftentimes the team members you are calling will not be happy that you are increasing their workload for the day and will ask for information to justify the consult. However, here are some tips that will allow you to call for a consult efficiently and confidently.

1. Know your patient's history very well. More often than not, after you call the subspecialty team members and explain the reason for the consult, they will have more questions for you. It is imperative that you know the patient very well to help answer these questions.

2. Know what question you are asking the consulting team. If you're going through the process of calling a consult, it

is because you have a specific question that you cannot answer. For example, what is the most appropriate antibiotic for the patient's pneumonia? This question should be clear before you attempt calling the consultant. If you have a clear question, the consultant will be better able to give you a clear answer.

3. Do not start the call by telling the consulting team members you are a medical student. This sounds a bit silly, but as long as you are clear as to the reason behind getting the consult and present the pertinent information, there is no need to tell them you are a medical student initially. Oftentimes just the fact that a medical student is calling them for a consult will be enough to make the consultant doubt your history and potentially even make him/her abrasive. Of course at the conclusion, you should give them your contact information and identify yourself as the medical student taking care of the patient.

The following is a format I liked to use when calling a consult. In this case, I'm a student on the pediatrics team calling the surgery team for a consult on a patient:

"Hello, this is Sujay Kansagra with the pediatrics team. We would like to get a surgery consult on one of our patients. The patient's name is John Doe in room 2526. His medical record number is 80001. The reason for consultation is to evaluate for possible appendicitis.

Briefly he is a twelve-year-old without any pertinent past medical history. He has had six hours of worsening right-sided lower abdominal pain. He has also had nausea and vomiting. His vitals are stable except for a fever of 39.2 and a heart rate of 120. His exam reveals rebound tenderness and guarding during abdominal exam, worse in the right lower quadrant. We performed an abdominal ultrasound, which shows some inflammation around his appendix. Anything else you would like to know? Great, how long do you think it will take until you see him? Once you've evaluated him, can you please page me? Again, I'm Sujay, the medical student taking care of him."

From the very beginning, I have given the consulting team all the necessary information to find the patient. I follow this by stating the reason we want them to evaluate the patient. This is followed by a very succinct history and physical exam that hopefully give the consulting team enough information to begin their assessment. Try to get some sense of how quickly the consulting team will see the patient and how they plan to communicate their plan with you. Leaving them with your pager number is always a good idea.

Chapter 35

How To Prepare for Shelf Exams

Most rotations finish with a test known as a shelf exam. It gets its name because the test consists of retired board questions that have been "shelved". It consists of multiple-choice questions that pertain to the rotation just completed. It is a standardized exam taken by students across the country and is created by the National Board of Medical Examiners (NBME). I found that the best way to prepare for the examination was to find a review book that I could read once or twice during the rotation, followed by doing as many practice questions as possible from question books. Most of the questions on a medical student shelf exam will pertain to the more important concepts within that particular field of medicine. Review books highlight those important topics, and question books will help engrain that knowledge. Of course patient care is also important in preparation for the shelf. Nothing helps a concept stick better than actually learning about a medical disorder by treating the patient.

The keys to doing well on the actual shelf exam are similar to keys for any standardized test. First it is very important to keep an eye on the clock. Avoid getting bogged down with specific questions that you do not know the answers to. Instead of obsessing for five minutes about a question, simply mark that question either on the answer sheet or the test itself so you know to come back to it. Chances are, if the answer is not apparent to you, obsessing over the next five minutes will not magically reveal the answer. Why waste precious time when you can always come back to this question later?

Another trick for questions that have long stems is to quickly look at the answer choices to get a sense of what type of question they will be asking. Will they be asking about the next step in the patient's workup? Are they asking for an actual diagnosis? Or is the question focusing on something completely different? By taking a quick look at the answer choices, you can actually read the question in the proper frame of mind. Don't waste time reading a long question and then getting to the answer choices and finding yourself going back through the entire question to find the pertinent information.

Finally remember that the shelf exam is only a portion of the rotation grade—and often a small portion. The most important thing is to do well while on the wards and be a productive part of the team. If you find that your time is limited, you should be focusing on reading about your patients rather than studying for the board exam.

Chapter 36

Teamwork

The importance of teamwork cannot be overemphasized. For the rest of your career, you'll be relying on a team of people to help take care of those who are ill. No one can do this job on his/her own. Even as a medical student, starting to think in the team mind-set is imperative. As previously mentioned, teamwork often factors into your rotation grade. The best way of showing that you are a team player is getting along with your fellow medical students during the rotation. As an attending, if I get the sense that a medical student is being overly competitive and trying to show themselves as superior over another student, he/she gets negative points in my book. Remember, a medical student should not answer questions that are directly addressed to another medical student unless the student appears to be asking for help. Never ever preround on patients who are not yours in hopes of getting an inside edge.

Not only is teamwork important among medical students, but also with the rest of the hospital staff. Nurses are an important part of your team, and you need to treat them as equals. Nurses truly can make or break your rotation experience. They are well aware that medical students are not proficient in clinical care. They can be a huge help to you in determining the next step for the patient and informing you of important clinical changes. Never approach a nurse with a sense of arrogance. They pick up on this quite quickly, and you will end up suffering the consequences.

The health unit coordinator (HUC) is the name given to the staff member who typically sits at the entrance to the inpatient floor and helps coordinate the logistics for admitted patients. This role may have a different name in your hospital. They are the ones who typically put charts together, keep track of which patients have left the floor, and inform nurses when there is a patient care need. This person often has a great deal of knowledge regarding the logistics of how the floor works. They can provide assistance if you have difficulty getting in touch with certain members of the hospital staff or even entering orders. Get to know your HUC.

Working as a team is not only the right thing to do for patient care, it will create a very healthy, happy working environment for you. Nothing is worse than coming into work and having coworkers with whom you do not get along. Those with increased stress in the work environment often carry that stress back home. Conflicts with other team members will interfere with your learning as a medical student and will end up reflecting on your evaluation. So remember that medicine is a team sport.

I hope these last few chapter have provided you with some guidance on how to approach the clinical rotations. It is a challenging year, but I encourage you to enjoy the learning process and avoid putting undue pressure on yourself. It is the only time in your medical career where you are not directly responsible for making decisions that affect patient care. You will always be supervised appropriately, so you should use this time to soak up everything you can about clinical medicine and appreciate your new role.

Chapter 37

Studying for the Boards

Students in allopathic medical schools pursuing MD degrees are required to take a series of United States Medical Licensing exams (USMLE). DO students are required to take a similar series of Comprehensive Osteopathic Medical Licensing Examinations (COMLEX), which is discussed later in this chapter, but often also take USMLE exams to open up options for residencies. Just hearing the term USMLE is enough to get a doctor's heart pumping. It brings back memories of intense studying and anxiety. It's another hurdle we must face in our journey to becoming doctors.

During the course of medical school and residency, allopathic students are required to complete four USMLE examinations. The first exam is known as Step 1 and consists of questions to test basic science knowledge. The next exam is Step 2 CK. This examination includes clinical scenarios that test knowledge acquired during rotations in medical school. The CK stands for clinical knowledge. The newest examination is Step 2 CS. The CS stands for clinical skills. This is an oral examination that is administered at only a handful of centers throughout the United States and overseas. It is meant to test a student's ability to adequately assess patients, conduct physical examinations, and then integrate knowledge from the history and physical to come up with a diagnostic plan and differential diagnosis for patients. The final exam is Step 3. This exam is similar to Step 2 CK in that it tests clinical knowledge. This examination is often completed during the first year of residency. It is a two-day examination.

The score for USMLE Step 1, 2 CK, and 3 is between 1 and 300. In 2016 the average score for USMLE Step 1, 2 CK, and 3 was 228, 242, and 225, respectively, while the passing score in 2017 was 194, 209, and 196, respectively. Approximately 5% of first-time test takers will fail the exam. If a student passes the examination, he/she is not allowed to repeat the exam. It is therefore crucial that students study as hard as possible so that they obtain the optimal score the first time.

Let's discuss each of these tests in turn, and go over strategies to acing your examinations.

USMLE Step 1

This examination is perhaps the most important for medical students. Although it was intended to ensure students understood the basic science concepts important to a medical knowledge foundation, residency programs use it widely to determine how suitable an applicant is for their residency program. For this reason medical students often study the hardest for this particular examination.

The material this examination covers is typically learned during the first two years of a traditional medical school curriculum. However, simply completing these courses in medical school is not enough preparation to do well on this examination. The material covered during medical school is often very detailed, and it is hard to remember the material once the course is over. Therefore this material needs to be reviewed again prior to the Step 1 examination. The test covers subjects such as pathology, pharmacology, physiology, microbiology, biochemistry, anatomy, and behavioral sciences.

The key to doing well on the Step 1 examination is essentially to memorize as much basic science information as one possibly can prior to the test. Because the test incorporates vast amounts of material, you should focus your studying on a high-yield source instead of trying to relearn the first two years of medical school. The review book most students use for Step 1 is known as *First Aid for the USMLE Step 1*. This book is a highly condensed overview of the main topics found in each of the basic science categories. I encourage all students to begin their preparation with this book. Not only should you read everything in the book, you should make an attempt to memorize every single small part of this book. The task can be a daunting one because the book covers a great deal of material. However, because this textbook tends to be very high yield, there is no sense in trying to learn material from other sources until you have completely memorized material from this book. I read the book multiple times, and then I made flash cards with every small piece of information I did not know. I then worked through the more than five hundred flash cards I had made, setting aside those cards that had material I had memorized. Unfortunately I had not learned my memory technique described in chapter 25 prior to taking Step 1. If I had known this technique, perhaps studying would have been much more efficient.

Although *First Aid* is a very useful resource for Step 1, it should be the start of your studying, not the totality. You will need to find other short review books to delve further into topics that *First Aid* may not have covered. I found *BRS Pathology* and *BRS Physiology* to be useful review books for those two subjects. I also used the book *Microbiology Made Ridiculously Simple*. I read each of these books at least two times. Finally I signed up for an online question bank. Many companies offer online questions for all of the board examinations. I used Kaplan Q-bank for Step 1. Access to online question banks can be expensive, but I still feel this is an important part of your preparation. Please note that most of the questions you will find in these question banks tend to be more specific than actual board questions. Don't be discouraged by the difficulty of these questions. They should *not* serve as a primary studying tool, but instead you should use them to gauge how well you're doing in your preparation. If I was getting 70 percent correct on my question bank tests, I was doing very well. Do not rely on question banks as the sole source of studying for a board examination.

The examination itself is conducted in certified testing centers, which are available in almost every major city in the United States. Your medical school should help guide you as far as when to take this exam. You would typically take it after the second year of medical school.

The examination itself is an eight-hour computerized exam. At the time this book was written, the test consisted of 280 multiple-choice questions divided into seven blocks. You must complete each block within an hour. Although there is a fifteen-minute orientation at the beginning of the examination, you should already be familiar with the format by taking a practice exam that is provided through the USMLE testing website (www.usmle.org/step-1).

You will find that the questions themselves vary as far as difficulty. Some are incredibly simple, while others are quite challenging. Questions may incorporate an audio or video component as well. Students have access to a table of normal values for various labs. You can refer to this table throughout the examination.

If there was ever an exam that you studied obsessively for, USMLE Step 1 should be that exam. Residency programs commonly use it to help choose residents. This may be the only board examination you have taken by the time you are applying to residency, so this score will be particularly important. It is imperative to put your best foot forward.

How long should you study for this exam? Although everybody looks for an answer to this question, nobody can tell you how long and hard you should study for this—or any other, for that matter—exam. Most students dedicate at least two months of preparation time, but the earlier you can start studying the better. Remember that if you start preparing very early, much of this earlier material will need review again leading up to the exam. You will also need to pace yourself so you do not burn out. Save the most intense studying for the few weeks leading up to the examination. During this time it is wise to go back to the high-yield books, such as *First Aid*, to ensure you know the core material.

Prior to arriving for the examination, you should recheck your testing site information and ensure you are bringing along the proper identification. Nothing is worse than studying for three months, only to show up and be turned away due to lack of proper ID. Drive to the location prior to the test date to determine exactly how to get there so you do not waste time the morning of the test. Just as with medical school interviews, you do not want to start the morning of the test worrying about how to get there and stressing out because you're running late.

So what are your chances of passing? Overall they are pretty good. In 2016 among first-time test takers in the United States and Canada, those pursuing an MD degree had a pass rate of 96 percent. Those pursuing a DO degree had a pass rate of 93 percent. Examinees who were not from US or Canadian schools had a pass rate of 78 percent if taking the test for the first time.

USMLE Step 2 CK

Although the USMLE Step 1 exam tends to be a very intense experience, the Step 2 CK examination is less stressful. The test is intended to determine clinical knowledge that students should gain during the core rotations in medical school. Test questions are typically presented in case presentation format. Similar to Step 1, the exam is conducted in a multiple-choice, computer-based format. The same testing centers that provide Step 1 testing conduct this test as well. The test itself is organized into eight blocks of questions at the time of writing this book. There are 318 questions in the entire exam. Students have one hour to complete each block. The examination time is nine hours.

Preparation for this examination tends to be less intense than for Step 1. Sometimes the scores from the Step 2 CK examination are not back prior to applying for residency. However, doing your best on this examination is still important because these scores may prove significant in applying for fellowships after residency. A variety of books provide nice reviews of the topics for the examination. My personal favorite is *Crush Step 2* by Brochert. Similar to Step 1, online question banks can be very useful in your preparation. I found USMLE World to be a good resource.

As far as overall studying time, students tend to study less than they did for Step 1. Common practice dictates that you should spend at least two weeks studying for this examination; however, in actuality, I would recommend spending a minimum of one month of daily studying.

The pass rate for Step 2 CK is similar to Step 1. For 2016 those pursuing an MD degree who took the test for the first time had a 97 percent passing rate. For those pursuing the DO degree, first-time test takers had a 94 percent pass rate. And for those who were not from US or Canadian schools, first-time takers had an 80 percent pass rate.

USMLE Step 2 CS

This board examination was implemented in 2004. It is the least convenient examination to take because it is only administered in five testing locations across the country, which are Atlanta, Chicago, Houston, Philadelphia, and Los Angeles. So in addition to the bank-breaking examination fees, students have to pay for travel to these locations. The test is designed to evaluate clinical skills by using a series of simulated patient encounters. Actors are hired to portray patients. During the examination, students complete twelve different patient encounters. Not all patient encounters will affect your score because a minority are pilot scenarios that they are testing for future exams.

You have fifteen minutes per encounter to take a history and physical. There won't be time to do a full history and physical. You must focus on relevant history and conduct a focused exam. After each patient interview is complete, you will be asked to write a note in ten minutes that includes history, physical exam, workup, and your differential diagnosis, with the top three possibilities and supporting evidence for each. Not all cases have a definite diagnosis, so don't feel you have missed something if a diagnosis doesn't jump out at you. If you finish examining the patient before fifteen minutes, you can add that remaining time to your ten minutes in which to write a note. Although the task seems daunting, this examination perhaps takes the least preparation of any of the board examinations. Regardless it is important not to blow off the examination completely.

To prepare for this examination, I read *First Aid for USMLE Step 2 CS*. It is not a particularly lengthy book. It provides the key points for the exam, such as remembering to wash your hands prior to examining the patient and asking the patient's permission to examine him/her. These are some simple steps that will help ensure you pass the examination.

Much like USMLE Step 2 CK, this exam has a very high pass rate. For MD-degree candidates taking the examination in 2016, there was a 97 percent pass rate for first-time test takers. For DO degree candidates, the pass rate was 91 percent. However, for applicants outside of the United States and Canada, the pass rate was 82 percent. Lack of proficiency in English does pose a significant disadvantage in this examination.

USMLE Step 3

This final examination is typically taken during the first year of residency. Similar to Step 2 CK, the purpose of this test is to use your clinical knowledge to answer questions in a case presentation format. This particular examination is a two-day test. The first day consists of six blocks of questions, for a total of about 235 multiple-choice questions over seven hours. This includes 60 minutes for each block and 60 minutes of break time. The second day is nine hours long. This day consists of 180 multiple-choice questions in six blocks, each lasting 45 minutes. This is followed by thirteen case simulations. The simulations are a very different testing format than what you are used to. Test takers read the case and then attempt to manage the patient in the simulation. Test takers actually enter orders and get various tests to determine the likely diagnosis. The simulation will move ahead in time by hours or days, give feedback on how the patient does, and ask further questions about workup. This format is particularly tricky; you should practice it thoroughly prior to the exam. The system itself is not intuitive to use. You can find a practice simulation online when you register. The importance of practicing these case scenarios cannot be overemphasized because this system can be hard to navigate.

Preparation for this examination is typically not too intense. Giving yourself a few weeks to review material from all of the core rotations in medical school is important. My book of choice for this examination is *Boards and Wards* by Ayala and Spellberg.

In 2016, the pass rate among first-time test takers was 96 percent for those pursuing MD degrees, 95 percent for DO degree test takers, and 86 percent for test takers not from the United States or Canada. Because this exam has no bearing on where you match for residency, students tend to take this test less seriously than the others. However, do note that when applying for fellowships, they will likely ask you for all of your board scores.

COMLEX

The COMLEX examinations for DO students are similar to the USMLE series. They consist of Level 1, Level 2-Cognitive Evaluation, Level 2-Performance Evaluation, and Level 3 exams. The first three exams are typically completed during medical school. The entire series roughly aligns with material tested in the USMLE series. For more information regarding format of each test, scores, and testing accommodations, please visit www.nbome.org. If you are a DO student, please talk to your advisor about whether it would be beneficial to take the USMLE series of examinations based on your career goals.

Becoming a fully licensed doctor has many hurdles, and the board examinations are just a few of these. The tests are another significant expense that drives many medical students deeper into debt. The fee schedule for 2018 is $610 to sit for USMLE Step 1 and Step 2 CK. The charge for USMLE Step 2 CS is $1,285. This figure does not include travel expenses. For USMLE Step 3, the fee is $850. This provides a nice segue into the topic of our next chapter—finances.

Chapter 38

Handling Your Finances

During medical training we learn how to manage blood sugar for those with diabetes. We learn how to manage uncontrolled hypertension and increased intracranial pressure. We are forced to learn how to manage our time. However, nowhere in medical training do they teach you about managing an important factor in determining your future quality of life—your finances.

Here is a sad reality: in 2017 the AAMC reported that the average medical school graduate left with about $250,000 of education debt. Although many students may believe that their future physician salaries will easily pay off debt in a short amount of time, the reality is often different. We often forget that although a $175,000 salary looks attractive, the IRS will take about 35 percent. Rent/mortgage, food, credit card bills, and interest on your student loans will also take their share. You won't have nearly as much money as you think to pay back student loan debt after accounting for these other expenses. Only after accumulating a mountain of this debt do many people realize that the medical profession does not lead to wealth and riches. In most situations, medicine provides for a relatively comfortable lifestyle, but it is far from the popular notion of a luxurious life. Realize this fact very early in your training so that you can budget appropriately and create a sensible plan for the future. Such a plan not only involves the basic concepts of minimizing student loan debt and living frugally, but also involves a better understanding of financial tools, such as retirement planning and knowledge of how the stock market works. In this chapter I will cover these important considerations to help you on the road to a healthy and happy financial future.

Debt Matters

The first and most important lesson I can teach you regarding financial health is that debt matters. The accumulation of debt during college and postgraduate education can plague you for many years to come. Let's do some math. The figure of $250,000 in debt does not include other forms of debt, such as car loans and credit cards. Let's assume an interest rate of 6.5 percent, a plan for a three-year residency during which you defer payment (but interest accrues), and then a salary of $175,000 per year. If you put 15 percent of a $175,000 salary toward your loan, you would pay it off in just under 15 years, with a total interest of $211,000. That's right—you actually end up paying almost double the amount of the original debt due to accrued interest. So even a small number like 6.5 percent interest can end up making a big difference in the long run.

This brings me to an important point about the financial world. Finances are just a big game of percentages, whether it be the percentage you are earning in your savings account, the percentage you owe on your loans, or the percentage of inflation every year. It's all about percentages. The quicker you can make the percentages work in your favor rather than against you, the better off you will be.

We have already discussed how even a number as small as 6 percent a year can make such a large difference in your overall debt repayment. In the financial world, 6 percent a year is a moderate percentage amount. If someone's stock market portfolio gains about 9 percent a year, that is considered a very good return. Most of the safer investments would get you much less than 9 percent. Most savings accounts at the time this book was written will give you less than 1 percent interest per year.

Another important percentage to keep in mind is inflation. What is inflation? Simply put, inflation means that the cost of products continues to increase over time, thus making the amount you can buy with a dollar less. So one hundred dollars today will get you much less twenty years in the future, just as it got you much more twenty years in the past. On average, inflation is about 3 percent each year. So that one dollar will get you 3 percent less each year as inflation increases. Having $10,000 stuffed in your mattress means you are essentially losing the value of your money each year because that same amount will get you less in the real world. You want your saved money growing every year, ideally by more than 3 percent.

Now that you have a sense of how percentages play such a big role in the financial world, you will have a better sense of why credit card debt is the worst possible thing you can do to yourself. According to Bankrate.com, the average credit card interest rate at the time of writing this book was about 16 percent! Let me repeat—16 percent! That number should frighten you. In the financial world, 16 percent is huge. Making 16 percent on any investment each year is incredibly hard, and yet credit card companies are able to make this kind of money from you.

They offer nice, low monthly payments, and you are tempted to continue putting off making full payments. But in doing this, you are committing financial suicide. Your credit card debt will quickly grow if you keep spending and making only minimal payments. If that new TV costs you $1,000, you put it on your credit card, and your initial minimal payment is only $20, it will take you more than ten years to pay off your $1,000 if you keep making minimal payments. And during this time, you will also have paid $994 in just interest. So that TV actually costed nearly double. And not just that, the extra $994 that you spent in interest could have been used to make *you* money in the stock market or in a savings account, so you've really ended up losing out on even more. I'm not saying credit cards are all bad. You should own some credit cards to build your credit score. Some do offer nice perks, and a few even give you cash back. But please pay down the *entire* balance *every single month* so no interest accrues. If you cannot do this, don't use credit cards. I cannot emphasize this enough.

Now that we've discussed how percentages can work against you in the long term, let's look at how percentages can work for you by teaching you about the stock market.

Introduction to the Stock Market

Many people find the stock market a bit intimidating. Don't be one of those people. Understanding the stock market is actually incredibly simple, and starting to invest is just as easy. Let me give you some basics to get started.

First, what is a stock? A stock is essentially a small part of the company. For example let's say there is a company called Exampitech. This company decides it wants to go public, which means it wants to sell shares of its company to the general public. It decides it will divide the company into a thousand shares. Therefore each share is worth 0.1% of the company. Because the value of the entire company is about $500,000, it decides to sell each share for $500, or 0.1% of the total value of the company. Follow me so far?

So who buys these shares? When a company goes public, anyone can buy these shares. The shares of a company are bought and sold by people through a marketplace known as the stock market. Appropriate name, huh? But you can't just walk up to the stock market, lay down some cash, and say, "Give me some shares of Exampitech." Instead, the buying and selling is done through an intermediary known as a brokerage house. The brokerage house takes your order and then buys the shares for you from the stock market.

So why would a company want to divide itself up and sell itself to lots of ordinary people? The answer is money, of course. When a company goes public, even though the company has a total of $500,000 worth of assets, and therefore one stock should be worth $500, people will typically pay much more. That's because they feel the company will start to make more money, and in a few years, might be worth $1 million. So instead of selling each share for $500 as we mentioned earlier, the company can sell its shares for $600, for example. The company can then use the extra money it gains from selling shares to make itself even bigger, thereby helping make even more money.

Thousands of companies have decided to go public, and you can buy their shares through brokerages. Most of these companies have divided themselves into millions, if not billions, of shares. People want to buy shares of companies they think will make money and grow because if they do, the share price will also grow. They can then sell their shares in the future and end up making money.

That is the ultimate goal of investing money in the stock market.

Each stock is assigned a symbol to make it easy to find. For example Ford has the symbol F, and Apple has the symbol AAPL. Some people get creative with the symbol. For example the symbol for Harley-Davidson is HOG. The symbol is simply an easy way to find the stock price for a particular company. Where can you go to figure out how much a stock is currently worth? Lots of places! Newspapers regularly publish how much a stock was worth when the stock market closed the day before. But that's the old-fashioned way of looking up stock prices. These days we use the Internet where there are a multitude of websites to find stock market prices. Here is your first exercise:

Exercise 1: Look up the price for Apple stock.

Let's go to www.cnbc.com. This is just one of the many websites that offers you information on stock prices, but it is my favorite. Other sites include Yahoo, CNN, and Bloomberg. It doesn't matter where you get the quote. They all report the same numbers. Okay, so now that you are on the website for CNBC, a popular source for financial news, you will be confronted by lots of info:

news stories, the Dow Jones index, and lots of other stuff. Let's ignore all of it. Simply find the box that says "Search Quotes" or "Enter Symbols." This is where you will type in the symbol for Apple. Remember that symbol is AAPL. Once you hit enter, it takes you to a screen dedicated to Apple's stock. You will see lots of numbers and charts, but the two main numbers you are looking for should be at the very top. The first number is the current price for Apple. On the day I wrote this chapter, that number was $190.24. Next to the stock price will be another number with an up or down arrow. This indicates whether the stock has moved up or down on that particular day and by how much. My screen shows a green, upward-pointing arrow with the number $3.37 next to it. The price of Apple stock increased by $3.37 that day. Next to that number will be a percentage. That is the percentage of the stock price that the stock has changed that day. So for me that number is +1.8 percent. The stock price of Apple has increased by 1.8 percent. If you are checking the price at the time the market is actually open (Monday through Friday from 9:30 a.m. to 4:00 p.m. Eastern Standard Time), then the price will be changing every few seconds. This change is based on many different factors, but most important is the demand for the stock at that particular time. If the company is doing well and has put out some great news, then more people will want to buy it and the price will go up, and vice versa.

If you don't know the symbol for a company, it is pretty easy to find. Let's try another exercise.

Exercise 2: Find the stock price for Microsoft.

Most websites will have a place for you to look up symbols. In CNBC simply type in Microsoft in the box that says "Search Quote." Doing this should take you to another page where it lists matching results for Microsoft, including recent news and matching stock symbols. Because Microsoft sells its shares in a variety of different stock markets around the world, it may be listed multiple times with multiple symbols. We want to find the symbol for the US stock market. Do you see it? Click on it, and away you should go to the page for information on Microsoft's stock. If you are having trouble, the symbol is MSFT.

Now that you are familiar with stocks and how to look up their prices, let's talk about bonds. Simply put, bonds are a small loan. Companies, governments, and a variety of other groups sell bonds to raise money. When you buy a bond from such a group, you are simply lending money to the company or government that sold you the bond. In return the company or government will give you a certain percentage of extra money. So if I bought a government bond, the government would agree to give me 3 percent each year on the money I lent them by buying the bond. The difference between a stock and a bond is that a stock is an actual piece of the company. So its price will change depending on how well the company does. A bond is not a part of the company. It's simply a small loan you are giving to an organization in exchange for more money later. Typically less risk is involved in bonds, and therefore there is also less chance of making a lot of money. This is an important concept in finance. The riskier the investment, the more chances you can make or lose a lot of money. Individual stocks tend to be a risky investment because their prices can fluctuate quite a bit day to day. Bonds are less risky. Putting money in a savings account has almost no risk, and therefore very little return. This is about all you need to know about bonds for the sake of this book.

So what about people who like the idea of stocks, but don't like the idea of risking a lot of money? This is where the concept of diversification comes in. Have you ever heard someone say, "Diversify your stock portfolio"? This simply means you should try to invest in different types of companies so that even if one company goes bankrupt or does poorly, you won't lose all of your money. But the opposite also holds if you divide your money up. If one company does very well and the rest stay stable, your overall investment won't increase dramatically in price. The larger the number of stocks you own in different companies that do totally different things, the more diversified you are. This brings us to our next topic—the mutual fund.

What exactly is a mutual fund? A mutual fund is simply a collection of different types of stocks that a person, known as the mutual fund manager, has picked. The manager picks stocks he/she thinks will do well. The manager then assigns a brand-new symbol that represents this particular collection of stocks. This makes it easy for me to give the manager my money, so that the manager can put my money into each of the selected stocks. If I buy shares of a mutual fund, I'm actually buying small amounts of every stock in that particular mutual fund. Many mutual funds hold not only stocks, but bonds and other investments as well. But the concept is the same. The mutual fund manager is trying to make other people money by taking their money and buying a variety of different things.

So what benefit does the mutual fund manager get for taking your money and putting it into his/her mutual fund? Each mutual fund manager charges you a fee to take your money and invest it for you. The percentage can vary quite a bit, but it is typically around 1–2 percent. So every year mutual fund managers take 1–2 percent of the money you have put into their hands and put it into their pockets. But that's not the only way they make money. Many mutual funds also charge a load, a term for a certain percentage they take up front or when you sell the mutual fund. A front-end load, which is taken at the initial time of investment, can be upwards of 5 percent. So right from the beginning, 5 percent of your money is gone, and the remaining 95 percent is invested in the mutual fund. These percentages can add up very quickly. But this is something that many investors don't mind paying because they feel the mutual fund manager knows best about which investments to buy, thereby making the investor more money.

Exercise 3: Find the price for a mutual fund.

The symbols for mutual funds are often five letters. Try typing in AMRMX, the symbol for a mutual fund by a company known as American Funds. The company offers a wide variety of different mutual funds, and this is just one example. The price you will see is for a share of the mutual fund, or essentially a piece of the mutual fund. The price fluctuates based on the prices of the various investments within the mutual fund. Try to click on the various tabs to find the expense ratio (hint, it's under "Profile"). This is the amount the company will charge you each year if you continue to own the mutual fund. You may also see the percentage the company charges as a load, either up front or as a back-end load (sometimes called a deferred load), which is charged if sell your shares of the mutual fund before a certain amount of time. These are all ways for the mutual fund manager to make money.

If you are a beginner in the stock market and don't feel as though you want to buy individual stocks, I would encourage you to check out mutual funds from Vanguard. Vanguard has a wide variety of mutual funds that charge very low fees. For example VTSMX is the Vanguard Total Stock Market Fund, which essentially is a very large mutual fund made up of stocks in just about every company in the American stock market. By buying a share of VTSMX, you have essentially bought a very small piece of every stock. As the stock market goes up or down, so does the price of a share of VTSMX. At the time of writing this book, its expense ratio was 0.15 percent (less than one-fifth of one percent), which is about as low as you can find. And this fund doesn't charge a load!

Exercise 4: Open a brokerage account.

Now that you know the basics of the stock market and realize that it is not as complicated as you may have thought, you might want to try to actually invest a small amount of money on your own to get some real-life experience. Fancy brokerage houses will help give you advice on which stocks to buy and do the buying and selling for you—all at a price. These days most young investors don't use this type of brokerage house. Instead they open up online accounts at a brokerage like Robinhood, Etrade or TDAmeritrade. By opening up an account, you have the ability to buy and sell shares of stocks on your own. The online brokerage takes your order electronically, sends it to the stock market, and then holds onto your stocks for you. Be sure to take the tutorials these websites offer before investing any real money. If you are interested in further reading about the stock market and investing, I strongly recommend the Motley Fool series of books, which have guidebooks for almost any level of investor. Start with the basic books first. And remember that if you make money by buying and then selling a stock, you will have to pay taxes on that gain. If you simply hold the stock, you do not have to pay taxes unless you sell it for a profit or unless the stock pays a dividend. A dividend is a small cash payment from the company for every share you own as a way of encouraging people to buy and hold their stock.

The important parts of your financial health don't stop here. This is just the start. Once you know how the stock market works, you can start to delve into the importance of retirement accounts. Research why an IRA (individual retirement account) is important. Look up the difference between a traditional IRA and Roth IRA. Take control of your finances by constantly increasing your financial knowledge. Don't let the stock market intimidate you. It's not that complicated after all.

Chapter 39

Your Health—Sleeping, Mood, Stress, and Diet

Doctors are great at taking care of other people. Unfortunately we often forget to take care of ourselves. And whether we like to believe it or not, neglecting our own health can potentially affect the care we provide for patients. The popular saying "Do as I say, not as I do" should not apply to doctors. We should exemplify the good health we wish to instill in our patients. With that in mind, this chapter is dedicated to ensuring that we stay healthy on our journey to becoming doctors.

Sleep

Do not skip over this section! If there is one thing I could go back and do differently, it would be to manage my sleep much better during college and medical school. I slept through the majority of my classes and had a great deal of difficulty staying awake with every attempt to study. Had I known what I do now about sleep, I would have been a more efficient student with better grades, more rest, and better health. I do not want you to make the same mistake.

Sleep and the medical field have never gotten along well. They appear to be in a constant battle. The medical field often views the concept of a full night's sleep as a luxury. Years of overnight call and the forty-eight-hour shift have led many to believe that doctors are somehow able to function without any sleep. This situation has also created a culture where many feel that sleep is for the weak and "I'll sleep when I die." Only recently has the field of medicine started putting more emphasis on sleep given the tie between resident fatigue and medical errors. Unfortunately many students still believe that they can get away with a minimal amount of sleep and continue functioning at their best. I myself was such a student. However, you should know some very interesting facts about sleep. By changing our attitudes toward sleep, I believe that each of us can become better, more efficient students and providers.

The first question that always comes up is how much sleep do you really need. This is different for each person. For adults the average amount of time needed to feel fully refreshed and function optimally is between seven and nine hours. In fact studies show that the average adult needs slightly over eight hours of sleep to feel completely refreshed. Some rare individuals truly need only six hours of sleep to function at the optimum. On the other side of the equation, there are also "long sleepers" who need upwards of ten hours to feel fully refreshed. But again, most adults fall within the seven-to-nine-hour range. Your sleep need is biologically set. You can do nothing to change your sleep need. Many people are under the false impression that they can get accustomed to smaller amounts of sleep. This unfortunately is not true. Studies show that the longer we are sleep-deprived, the less we are able to perceive how sleepy we are. So people can be tricked into thinking they have gotten used to sleeping shorter periods of time. However, if the same sleep-deprived person undergoes objective testing of alertness and vigilance, performance will continue to worsen the longer he/she is sleep-deprived. So even though you may feel that you have gotten accustomed to sleeping only six hours, objective data show that this is not the case. So my first piece of health advice—and perhaps the most important—is to get adequate sleep. This is usually around eight hours, but it varies depending on the person.

Many will read this suggestion and think, "How can I possibly get eight hours of sleep? After all, I have lots of work and studying to do, and this can't be done without staying up late at night, right?" Wrong.

Let me take you back to my undergraduate experience. During my junior year, I convinced myself that I needed only six hours of sleep every single night. I did not feel particularly tired upon waking up each morning, and therefore figured I was still getting an adequate amount of sleep. However, for almost all of my classes, I would fall asleep within the first ten minutes of lecture. The remainder of the class was spent in a semi-daze, trying to keep my eyes open. I would make up for this lack of learning during class by studying extra hard outside of the classroom. I would often need to stay up late prior to exams to study the material. However, every time I tried to study, I would also be similarly tired and constantly fall asleep while reading the material. As you can imagine, this was a very inefficient way of learning anything. Not only was my time in the classroom wasted, the studying outside of class took much longer than it should have due to my constant fatigue and sleepiness. Combine this with the fact that sleep is incredibly important for memories and learning, and you're left with a very inefficient student. So although you may feel it's necessary to stay up late and skip out on sleep to get extra work done, chances are you're much less efficient due to your sleep deprivation. So you might be "wasting" one or two hours by sleeping extra, however, if you are 50 percent more efficient during the day, then you are still getting much more work done in a shorter time. So sleeping more is a win-win. You do better in school and feel much less fatigued throughout the day.

But wait, can't you just drink lots of caffeine to stay awake? Many people do use caffeine as a drug to get by with less sleep. However, although you may not be feeling the effects of caffeine at nighttime, chances are the caffeine you consume in your day is still floating around in your bloodstream at bedtime. Your body gets rid of half the caffeine in your system every three to seven hours. So even some of your morning caffeine intake will be in your system at night. Caffeine disrupts sleep. It causes less deep sleep, and therefore your nighttime sleep might not be as refreshing. This of course leads to more caffeine intake the next day to make up for the fact that you slept poorly the night before. This is a great cycle for the coffeemakers but a terrible thing for you. So get out of the coffee/poor sleep/more coffee circle. Do not use caffeine as a drug to skip out on sleep. Give your brain what it needs, which is adequate amounts of rest.

How exactly can you figure out what your true sleep need is? This can be very difficult if you are chronically sleep-deprived. Chances are you have built up a sleep debt. Sleep debt is a very real thing. If you are chronically getting less sleep than you biologically need, your body needs payback for the sleep you have missed. Thankfully you do not need to pay back missed sleep one for one. So if you have denied yourself about two hours of sleep every night for the past five years, you do not necessarily have to pay back that much sleep. However, you will have to sleep more than your baseline sleep need for a consistent time to start feeling fully refreshed. I usually recommend students try to pay back the sleep debt during a holiday. This may entail sleeping for an excess of ten hours every night. Gradually you will find that you are not falling asleep the minute your head hits the pillow, and you are waking up on your own after less time asleep. Ideally you will end up requiring between seven and nine hours each night and will still be able to wake up feeling refreshed. The main indicators that you are caught up on your sleep debt and are getting adequate sleep are how you feel upon awakening and a lack of drowsiness during the day. Waking up in the morning should not be difficult if you've had adequate rest the night before. Once you figure out how many hours you need, continue to plan your day such that you are getting this adequate opportunity to sleep.

Now that we've discussed the importance of sleep and getting the right amount, let's tackle some of the other common sleep complaints that medical students have.

"I Can't Fall Asleep at Night"

This is a common complaint among medical students and the general population. Here are some things to try:

1. Improve your sleep hygiene. Sleep hygiene refers to the behaviors and environmental factors that may promote or disrupt sleep. The key aspects of good sleep hygiene include having a set bedtime and wake time. Keeping these consistent during both the weekdays and weekends is important. The next step is to avoid substances that can disrupt sleep, such as excessive caffeine and alcohol abuse. Third, it is important to avoid excessive light exposure at nighttime, such as from TVs, smartphones, and laptop

computers, as this artificial light will decrease your brain's natural melatonin synthesis, thereby disrupting sleep. Fourth, develop a nighttime routine that is performed the same way leading up to bedtime. This makes the transition to sleep easier and quicker. Keep the temperature on the cool side (68-72 degrees Fahrenheit), as your body temperature drops when you sleep and cool temperatures can help promote this drop.

2. Exercise during the day can be beneficial to nighttime sleep. However, avoid excessive exercise late in the evening or at night, as this raises your body temperature for a long time and makes it more difficult to fall asleep.

3. A hot nighttime shower artificially raises your body temperature and then causes a rapid drop. This can be advantageous to sleep onset. So consider a hot shower just before bedtime.

4. If you are the type of person who cannot seem to turn off your mind while you are lying in bed and are constantly thinking and worrying about sleep, you fall into a group of people known as psychophysiological insomniacs. This is a very common cause of insomnia.

The main problem is that your bed has become a place where you think and worry instead of a place where you sleep. Even people who are very tired can't seem to shut their brains off and finally go to sleep. To help treat this type of insomnia, sleep hygiene as discussed above is important as a foundation. However, the next step is trying to associate your bed and your bedroom only with sleep. That means you should do all of your other activities outside of your room and only use your bedroom for sleep.

Next you should attempt to break the association of excessive worry with your bedroom. Therefore if you're lying in bed for more than twenty minutes and find yourself worrying and thinking instead of sleeping, get out of your bed and do something boring (like reading). Then come back into bed only when you are sleepy. For those who are frequent clock checkers, I recommend turning the clock around or getting rid of the clock altogether. Medications for sleep and substances like alcohol are merely short-term fixes and not adequate long-term treatments for insomnia. They can also be dangerous and worsen sleep quality. You may want to consult your physician about your problem and ask for a referral to a sleep specialist. This book is not a substitute for professional medical help.

5. For those who are light sleepers, strongly consider buying foam earplugs. They are fairly cheap and can be found in any pharmacy. It is a good way to avoid excessive noise for those who live with roommates or have a loud neighborhood.

Stress

We all encounter stress in our daily lives. A small amount of stress can be a good thing, as it motivates us to work hard and study. However, excessive stress can be counterproductive. Here are some tricks to keeping stress at a manageable level.

1. Exercise regularly. Even a small amount of exercise each day can help lift your mood and relieve stress.

2. Find time for activities you enjoy. You should not feel guilty for taking some time away from studying. Having time to relax may make you a more efficient learner.

3. Make a list. If you only have one or two things to get done, you don't need a list. But as this number grows, our brains play a funny trick on us. We begin to feel

that there is a lot more to get done than there actually is. There were times when I felt overwhelmed due to the false belief that I had seven or eight things to get done, but when I wrote them out, there were only four or five items on the list. So make a list. It makes everything seem more manageable. And there is no greater feeling than being able to cross through an item on the list when it's done.

4. Keep things in perspective. The younger you are, the more likely you are to feel that your grades are everything. Granted they are very important, but there is much more to life (and much more to being successful in school) than just grades. As you get older, the more you will appreciate life outside of the bubble that is schoolwork.

5. Try to change your mentality about work. In medical school studying became something I actually enjoyed doing. I felt that every minute I spent working I was getting further and further ahead. This was very satisfying to me, and studying became something I wanted to do, not something I had to do. This allowed me to tolerate the workload much better and not get too stressed.

6. Add a little boogey. It's hard to be stressed while listening to your favorite music.

7. Get some sun. Sunlight can boost your mood and energize you. Take some time to play outside.

8. Avoid the drama. Nothing adds stress to your life like bad relationships with peers and significant others. Be smart about who you choose to associate with.

9. Be your own best friend. It's okay if you don't have a tight group of friends in medical school. Oftentimes school can be a bit isolating. You should still do things that make you happy, and it's okay to do them by yourself.

Depression and Anxiety

Both of these are quite common in medical school. After all, you are in a brand-new environment, often away from friends and family, with a huge workload and a great deal of pressure. You should realize that you are far from alone. Seek appropriate help if you feel that your mood or anxiety is interfering with your life. All schools have health services through which to get the appropriate help.

Diet

Fight the temptation to skip meals or eat out every night. Take time to hit the grocery store and do some cooking. Not only will it save you plenty of cash, but you will be a healthier and more energetic person for it. And because you will be spending lots of time during medical school in a rather sedentary lifestyle due to the workload, it is especially vital to avoid unhealthy foods.

I hope this chapter has convinced you on the importance of your health. You will find it difficult to take care of others if you haven't taken care of yourself first. Here is a checklist of the main points:

Dr. K's Checklist for Staying Healthy

☐ Don't cheat on sleep. The average adult needs seven to nine hours per night.

☐ Avoid abusing caffeine. A good night's sleep has no substitute.

☐ Find effective ways to reduce stress—exercise, get sunlight, eat healthy, and avoid social drama.

☐ Acknowledge that anxiety and depression are common. Seek help if they are affecting your life.

Chapter 40

Staying Human, Avoiding the Jade

Most residents can tell you that at some point in their medical training, they stopped acting like humans and instead acted more like robots. These robots would go about their daily assignments as quickly as possible, cut conversations with patients short, and refer to cases as the "same old, same old." This robotic state leads to a lack of satisfaction for the residents and poor patient rapport. But how can you avoid becoming desensitized to the cases you see after months and months of dealing with patients as a medical student?

I encourage you to take note of how you felt when you first started working on the wards in your hospital. Remember the awe and wonder you felt about medicine. Remember the nervousness you had examining your first patient. Remind yourself of these feelings when cases start becoming routine. Most importantly don't treat any patient as just another case. Remember that patient is someone's mother, or brother, or child. Treat your patients the same way you want others to treat your family members. Give them your time and attention. The goal of your workday should not be getting home. The goal should always be taking care of others. Keep this goal at the forefront through your entire medical career, and I promise you will have a more satisfying and rewarding life in medicine.

Also remember that a routine case for you may be the worst day of the patient's and family's life. Understand that patients and their families feel a great deal of stress, even for cases you may not find medically challenging. Acknowledging this concern and respecting how they are feeling is important. Never make a family feel like you have much sicker patients to worry about. Everyone should feel listened to and well treated.

If you still feel yourself becoming desensitized to taking care of patients, I recommend seeing your own doctor for a checkup. Not only is it important to maintain your own health, but it's important to become the patient every now and then. Being the patient makes us feel vulnerable, nervous, and sometimes frightened. Keep this feeling in mind when you see patients in the hospital who are acutely ill and have all of those feelings multiplied a thousand-fold.

Chapter 41

Applying for Residency

At the end of every successful medical school career comes the time to choose a field of medicine. This specialized training is known as residency. It can be a very easy decision for some students but a very challenging decision for many others. This chapter is dedicated to assisting you pick a specialty that's right for you and helping you navigate through the process of matching into a residency program.

What Type of Doctor Should I Be?

This is a common question. Many aspects go into deciding on a residency and career. If you are not already set on a certain path, the main way to help narrow down your choices is by exposing yourself to as many different specialties as possible. This process is easy to do for the core specialties because most medical students rotate through these programs during the third year of medical school. However, for those of you who are interested in a smaller branch of medicine, such as pathology or radiology, you might have limited exposure during your third year, and by the time fourth year rolls around, it is already time to decide and apply. Fortunately, many schools allow dedicated time during third year for elective rotations in these smaller fields. Explore your interests during these electives.

If you still have trouble deciding even after exposing yourself to a variety of fields, you can try using some online tools to narrow down the choices. Visit aamc.org and search for "Careers in Medicine." Once registered on the site, you are able to narrow down your choices by identifying your interests in medicine, your lifestyle goals, and other contributing factors.

Here is a useful chart to get you started, which has some of the most common residencies. I've listed the number of years necessary to complete training. I've also included the number of US applicants and number of available spots from the 2017 match process, which are directly from the National Residency Match Program (NRMP). At the end of the chart, I've created my own "competitive index" by dividing the number of applicants by the number of available spots. The higher the number, the higher the proportion of students who are competing for fewer spots. The most competitive residencies include plastic surgery, orthopedic surgery, dermatology, radiology, neurosurgery, otolaryngology, and general surgery.

RESIDENCY	Years of Training	# of US Applicants	Available Spots	Competitive Index
Anesthesiology	4#	1075	1202	0.9
Child Neurology	5	118	128	0.9
Dermatology	4#	479	423	1.1
Diagnostic Radiology	5#	909	932	1.0
Emergency Medicine	3 - 4	1845	2047	0.9
Family Practice	3	1797	3356	0.5
General Surgery	5	1382	1281	1.1
Internal Medicine	3	3837	7233	0.5
Internal Medicine/ Pediatrics	4	342	381	0.9
Neurological Surgery	6*	218	212	1.0
Neurology	4#	451	492	0.9
OBGYN	4	1202	1288	0.9
Orthopedic Surgery	5*	845	727	1.2
Otolaryngology	5	303	305	1.0
Pathology	4	232	601	0.4
Pediatrics	3	2056	2738	0.8
Plastic Surgery	6	200	159	1.3
Psychiatry	4	1067	1495	0.7
Radiation Oncology	5#	177	204	0.9

*Includes one year of general surgery.

#Includes one transitional/preliminary year.

How to Get the Residency You Want

The same concepts that applied for college and medical school admissions apply to residency. For example, grades and standardized test scores once again make up the core of your application. Many medical schools rank their students, so where you fall will be considered. Your test scores on the USMLE exams, particularly Step 1, are also very important.

After these two core components, the next most important aspect is once again your extracurriculars. Taking time to participate in activities during medical school is important. Certain activities tend to stand out when applying to residency. Research is one such activity, particularly for more competitive residencies. Publishing a research article in a scientific journal is perhaps the most impressive single thing you can do apart from great grades and test scores.

You also need letters of recommendations, so try to get to know some faculty well. Work closely with faculty in the particular field to which you are applying. They will not only help with recommendations, but they can serve as mentors and help open up doors in the future.

At this point in your career, I would say that your interview is just as important as your application. The further you get in training, the more important your personality and demeanor will be for those making the selections. As a resident, your ability to work with the team and get along with faculty can really bolster or hurt a residency program. So programs are not just looking for those who are good on paper, but also for the personable, hardworking people who will make good residents.

Let's discuss the process that residents go through to get a residency spot.

Steps to Getting a Residency

The process of applying for residency can be labor intensive and stressful. But hopefully when all is said and done, you will end up with a great residency spot. This section describes the application process for those interested in programs accredited by the Accreditation Council for Graduate Medical Education (ACGME). Students who graduate with an MD or DO degree can apply for these spots. In addition to ACGME programs, DO graduates can also apply to programs accredited by the American Osteopathic Association (AOA). This process is not discussed in this chapter but more information can be found at www.natmatch.com/aoairp. Check with your school for more details regarding this option.

The application process begins with the Electronic Residency Application Service (ERAS) for most residencies. At the time of writing this book, the exceptions were ophthalmology and some plastic surgery programs who use the San Francisco Match (sfmatch.org). Please check with your school's advisory program or online for the most up-to-date information.

ERAS is a centralized application service run by the AAMC that allows you to submit your residency application to almost any residency program you desire. Consider it similar to the Common Application for college. It also holds your letters of recommendation and your board scores, which are then sent out as one residency application. Applicants should have completed USMLE Step 1.

Once your ERAS application is complete, you will have to decide to which residency programs to send your application. Some apply to only a few (five or six), while others apply to more than twenty-five. It really depends on the strength of your application and the competitiveness of your specialty. Try to narrow down your choices as much as possible given the expense of applying and traveling to different programs. But be sure to apply to enough so that you feel confident you will find a residency spot. A great tool to help you is AAMC's "Apply Smart to Residency".

This website gives you useful strategies in the application process and helps you determine the right number of programs to which to apply based on your board scores and specialty.

Once your application is filled and sent to programs, you will hopefully be invited to interview.

Finally once you have interviewed at the programs that were interested in your application, you then have to apply to the National Residency Matching Program (NRMP). The NRMP is a service that matches medical students to residency programs. This is called the Residency Match. You will submit a list of residency programs where you interviewed, ranked in order from your top choice to last choice. You do not have to rank every program where you interviewed, only those in which you would want to train. The individual residency programs also turn in their list of top candidates from best to worst. Programs may decide not to include certain applicants who interviewed on their rank list if deemed unqualified for their program. The NRMP then matches students to residency programs based on these lists. It is incredibly important to realize that the match is a student-favored process. If a student ranks a program number one, and the program ranks the student high enough on their list such that there is an available spot, then the student will get that spot. *This means you should rank your schools in the order you liked the programs, not the order you feel programs are likely to rank you.* Even though you reach for a very competitive program and rank it number one, and that program doesn't choose you, it doesn't decrease your chances of matching at your number-two choice. So please remember this when you make your list of choices.

Once students and residents have turned in their lists, everyone is matched up. At the beginning of Match Week, students get an email telling them if they matched, but does not say to which program. For students who did not match at any program, there is a second round of matching over the next few days known as the Supplemental Offer and Acceptance Program (SOAP). Through SOAP, residency programs that did not fill their spots offer them to students who did not match. At the end of the process, almost everyone should be matched up somewhere. At the end of Match Week comes Match Day, a culminating event in the life of a medical student, during which the entire class finds out where they matched. To understand fully the emotion and excitement (and sometimes the disappointment) that comes with this day, I encourage you to read the chapter called "The Match" in my medical school memoir, *Everything I Learned in Medical School.*

So, to summarize the steps in finding a residency for allopathic medical students:

Step 1: Decide what type of doctor you want to be.

Step 2: Complete at least USMLE Step 1.

Step 3: Submit application via ERAS (mid-September).

Step 4: Interview at various residency programs.

Step 5: Submit your rank list via NRMP (deadline mid-February).

Step 6: Celebrate on Match Day (mid-March)

Choosing the Right Residency Program

So many factors go into deciding on a residency program that's right for you. Here are a few factors to consider:

1. Location of the program
2. Reputation of the program
3. Size of the program
4. Cost of living
5. Diversity of the patient population
6. Housestaff morale
7. Entertainment opportunities outside of the hospital
8. Call schedule
9. Salary
10. Vacation time

11. Research opportunities

12. Work/life balance

This list is far from inclusive of all the aspects that go into deciding on the best program for you. Many people report a "feeling" they get when they visit the right residency program for them. Don't ignore this feeling. Sometimes the gut knows best.

International Applicants

Foreign medical graduates (FMGs) often find success in trying to obtain medical residency spots in the United States. The process can be different depending on your country's rules. I encourage all applicants outside of the United States and Canada to visit ECFMG.org, which provides you with a great deal of material to help manage the journey. Here are a few recommendations to increase your chances of acceptance in a US residency program.

1. Try to spend some time working in a US hospital. Even if it means doing an observership, try to get some clinical exposure in the United States. Not only will doing so make you more comfortable with the US medical system, it will also provide you with possible recommendation letters.

2. Do a US rotation. If your medical school has ties with schools in the United States, try to do a formal rotation here. Residency programs want to ensure you can cut it in the US environment, and you have no better way to prove it than by doing well in a rotation in the United States.

3. Practice the language. One important consideration for residency programs is how well residents are able to communicate. This is especially important in medicine, where communication between patient and doctor, and between doctors, is so vital. Take time to practice English as much as possible so programs don't overlook you due to the language barrier.

Chapter 42

The Next Step After Residency—Private Practice versus Academic Medicine

Your career decisions do not end after choosing a specialty. Perhaps one of the most important choices you will make is whether to go into academic medicine or private practice. This chapter provides a quick overview of what each type of medicine entails to help you make a more informed decision.

Academic medicine is what each resident is most familiar with at the conclusion of training. The goals of academic medicine are to teach medical students and residents, as well as conduct research to help advance the field of medicine. Therefore you would practice academic medicine at large teaching institutions. Academic medicine careers tend to be somewhat less rigorous when it comes to overall number of hours spent with patients. This of course varies substantially based on the individual; however, the overall trend is that the academic medicine lifestyle is much more flexible. Physicians are typically given time each week dedicated to research, teaching, or administrative roles. Therefore they do not spend every single day in clinic seeing patients. Academic institutions do tend to attract the more difficult subspecialty cases because these institutions have more specialized physicians.

Private practice physicians are not typically involved in teaching or research of any kind. Their primary goal is to see patients. Because private practice physicians spend more time seeing patients, they also tend to generate more revenue and therefore tend to have higher salaries. However, they also tend to be under more pressure to generate a certain amount of revenue for the private practice group. Therefore these physicians tend to spend more time at work.

The most important thing is determining what you will enjoy for the rest of your life. Some people enjoy the variety that comes along with an academic career. However, others are dedicated to seeing patients and enjoy the higher compensation that comes along with private practice. There is no wrong decision regardless of what people may tell you. Choose what works best for you and your family.

Chapter 43

Closing

I hope this book has provided you with guidance. Please remember that the road to becoming a doctor will not be an easy one. Nobody ever said a life in medicine would be without challenges. You may run into ill-tempered people who will try to break your spirit. You will have to make sacrifices. You may experience self-doubt and anxiety. Although we might not talk about it, we all share similar experiences and struggles from time to time. But always keep in mind the reason you went into medicine in the first place. In a world filled with greed, hatred, and people who want to destroy, you have dedicated your life to healing and compassion. It is the noblest of callings. So no matter the challenges a life in medicine may bring, so long as you stay true to your patients and to yourself, you will never go wrong. Good luck.

Appendix A:
Common Medical Abbreviations

A&O: Alert and oriented

A/P: assessment and plan

ABG: arterial blood gas

AMA: against medical advice

ANA: antinuclear antibody

ARF: acute renal failure

BID: bi-daily, or twice a day. Commonly written on prescriptions when medication should be taken twice daily

BKA: below the knee amputation

BMP: basic metabolic profile (includes sodium, potassium, chloride, bicarbonate, blood urea nitrogen, creatinine, and glucose)

BP: blood pressure

BUN: blood urea nitrogen

Bx: biopsy

CAD: coronary artery disease

CABG: coronary artery bypass graft

CBC: complete blood count

CC: chief complaint

Chem7: another name for BMP

CHF: congestive heart failure

CMP: complete metabolic profile

CNS: central nervous system

COPD: chronic obstructive pulmonary disease

Cr: creatinine

CRF: chronic renal failure

CSF: cerebrospinal fluid

CT: computerized tomography (a type of radiology scan)

CVA: cerebrovascular accident (aka stroke) or costovertebral angle

Cx: culture

CXR: chest x-ray

D/C: discontinue or discharge

DDx: differential diagnosis

DKA: diabetic ketoacidosis

DM: diabetes mellitus. DM1 is type 1 diabetes, DM2 is type 2

DNR: do not resuscitate

DVT: deep venous thrombosis

Dx: diagnosis

ECG or EKG: electrocardiogram

ENT: ear, nose and throat

ESR: erythrocyte sedimentation rate

EtOH: ethanol

ETT: endotracheal tube

FH or Fam Hx: Family history

FTT: failure to thrive

F/u: follow-up

Gtt: drops/drip (Latin for drop is "guttae") or glucose tolerance test

HA: headache

HCG: human chorionic gonadotropin

HCT: hematocrit

HEENT: head, eyes, ear, nose, and throat

Hg or Hgb: hemoglobin

HPI: history of present illness

HTN: hypertension

Hx: history. For example, patient has a hx of diabetes

IM: intramuscular

IO: intraosseous

IV: intravenous

JVD: jugular venous distention

KVO: keep vein open (IV fluids are often run at a slow rate just to keep the IV from clotting off)

LFT: liver function test

LOC: loss of consciousness

LP: lumbar puncture

LVH: left ventricular hypertrophy

Lytes: short for "electrolytes"

MAP: mean arterial pressure

Mg: milligram or magnesium

MI: myocardial infarction
MRI: magnetic resonance imaging
MRSA: methicillin resistant staphylococcus aureus
MVC: motor vehicle collision
NKDA: no known drug allergies
NPO: "nil per os" which is Latin for "nothing by mouth". It
means the patient should not be eating or drinking.
NSAID: non-steroidal anti-inflammatory drugs. e.g. Ibuprofen
qD or qdaily: every day
q8h: every 8 hours
QID: four times a day
QOD: every other day
OSA: obstructive sleep apnea
PE: pulmonary embolus or physical exam
PFT: pulmonary function test
PT: physical therapy or prothrombin time
PTT: partial thromboplastin time
PVC: premature ventricular contraction
ROS: review of systems
SLE: systemic lupus erythematosus
SOB: shortness of breath
SQ: subcutaneously
SVD: spontaneous vaginal delivery
SVT: supraventricular tachycardia
Sx: symptoms
TB: tuberculosis
TIA: transient ischemic attack
TID: Three times daily
TFT: thyroid function test
TSH: thyroid stimulating hormone
Tx: treatment or transplant
U/A: urinalysis
URI: upper respiratory infection
UTI: urinary tract infection
VBG: venous blood gas
WBC: white blood count or white blood cell
WNL: within normal limits

Appendix B:
List of Allopathic Medical Schools

Alabama
University of Alabama School of Medicine (Birmingham)
University of South Alabama College of Medicine (Mobile)

Arizona
University of Arizona College of Medicine (Tucson)
University of Arizona College of Medicine (Phoenix)

Arkansas
University of Arkansas for Medical Sciences College of Medicine (Little Rock)

California
Keck School of Medicine - University of Southern California (LA)
Loma Linda University School of Medicine (Loma Linda)
Stanford University School of Medicine (Stanford)
University of California, Davis, School of Medicine (Sacramento)
University of California, Irvine, School of Medicine (Irvine)
University of California, Los Angeles David Geffen School of Medicine (LA)
University of California, Riverside School of Medicine (Riverside)
University of California, San Diego School of Medicine (La Jolla)
University of California, San Francisco, School of Medicine (San Francisco)

Colorado
University of Colorado School of Medicine (Aurora)

Connecticut
University of Connecticut School of Medicine (Farmington)
Yale University School of Medicine (New Haven)

District of Columbia
George Washington University School of Medicine and Health Sciences
Georgetown University School of Medicine
Howard University College of Medicine

Florida
Charles E. Schmidt College of Medicine at Florida Atlantic University (Boca Raton)
Florida International University Herbert Wertheim College of Medicine (Miami)
Florida State University College of Medicine (Tallahassee)
USF Health Morsani College of Medicine (Tampa)
University of Central Florida College of Medicine (Orlando)
University of Florida College of Medicine (Gainesville)
University of Miami Leonard M. Miller School of Medicine (Miami)

Georgia
Emory University School of Medicine (Atlanta)
Medical College of Georgia at Georgia Regents University (Augusta)
Mercer University School of Medicine (Macon)
Morehouse School of Medicine (Atlanta)

Hawaii
University of Hawaii, John A. Burns School of Medicine (Honolulu)

Illinois

Chicago Medical School at Franklin Univ. of Medicine & Science (Chicago)
Loyola University Chicago Stritch School of Medicine (Maywood)
Northwestern University - Feinberg School of Medicine (Chicago)
Rush Medical College of Rush University Medical Center (Chicago)
Southern Illinois University School of Medicine (Springfield)
University of Chicago - Pritzker School of Medicine (Chicago)
University of Illinois College of Medicine (Chicago)

Indiana
Indiana University School of Medicine (Indianapolis)

Iowa
University of Iowa Roy J. and Lucille A. Carver College of Medicine (Iowa City)

Kansas
University of Kansas School of Medicine (Kansas City)

Kentucky
University of Kentucky College of Medicine (Lexington)
University of Louisville School of Medicine (Louisville)

Louisiana
Louisiana State University School of Medicine in New Orleans (New Orleans)
Louisiana State University School of Medicine in Shreveport (Shreveport)
Tulane University School of Medicine (New Orleans)

Maryland
Johns Hopkins University School of Medicine (Baltimore)
Uniformed Services University of the Health Sciences F. Edward (Bethesda)
University of Maryland School of Medicine (Baltimore)

Massachusetts
Boston University School of Medicine (Boston)
Harvard Medical School (Boston)
Tufts University School of Medicine (Boston)
University of Massachusetts Medical School (Worcester)

Michigan
Central Michigan University College of Medicine (Mount Pleasant)
Michigan State University College of Human Medicine (East Lansing)
Michigan State University College of Human Medicine (Midland)
Oakland University William Beaumont School of Medicine (Rochester)
University of Michigan Medical School (Ann Arbor)
Wayne State University School of Medicine (Detroit)

Minnesota
Mayo Medical School (Rochester)
University of Minnesota Medical School (Minneapolis)

Mississippi
University of Mississippi School of Medicine (Jackson)

Missouri
Saint Louis University School of Medicine (St. Louis)
University of Missouri-Columbia School of Medicine (Columbia)
University of Missouri-Kansas City School of Medicine (Kansas City)
Washington University in St. Louis School of Medicine (St. Louis)

Nebraska
Creighton University School of Medicine (Omaha)

University of Nebraska College of Medicine (Omaha)
Nevada
University of Nevada School of Medicine (Reno)
New Hampshire
Geisel School of Medicine at Dartmouth (Hanover)
New Jersey
Cooper Medical School of Rowan University (Camden)
University of Medicine and Dentistry of NJ- NJ Medical School (Newark)
University of Medicine and Dentistry of New Jersey-Robert Wood Johnson Medical School (Piscataway)
New Mexico
University of New Mexico School of Medicine (Albuquerque)
New York
Albany Medical College (Albany)
Albert Einstein College of Medicine of Yeshiva University (Bronx)
Columbia University College of Physicians and Surgeons (New York)
Hofstra North Shore - LIJ School of Medicine (Hempstead)
Icahn School of Medicine at Mount Sinai (New York)
New York Medical College (Valhalla)
New York University School of Medicine (New York)
State University of New York Downstate Medical Center (Brooklyn)
State University of New York Upstate Medical University (Syracuse)
Stony Brook University School of Medicine (Stony Brook)
University at Buffalo State University of New York School of Medicine & Biomedical Sciences (Buffalo)
University of Rochester School of Medicine and Dentistry (Rochester)
Weill Cornell Medical College (New York)
North Carolina
Duke University School of Medicine (Durham)
The Brody School of Medicine at East Carolina University (Greenville)
University of North Carolina at Chapel Hill School of Medicine (Chapel Hill)
Wake Forest School of Medicine Baptist Medical Center (Winston-Salem)
North Dakota
Univ. of North Dakota School of Medicine and Health Sciences (Grand Forks)
Ohio
Case Western Reserve University School of Medicine (Cleveland)
Northeast Ohio Medical University (Rootstown)
Ohio State University College of Medicine (Columbus)
The University of Toledo College of Medicine (Toledo)
University of Cincinnati College of Medicine (Cincinnati)
Wright State University Boonshoft School of Medicine (Dayton)
Oklahoma
University of Oklahoma College of Medicine (Oklahoma City)
Oregon
Oregon Health & Science University School of Medicine (Portland)
Pennsylvania
Drexel University College of Medicine (Philadelphia)
Jefferson Medical College of Thomas Jefferson University (Philadelphia)

Pennsylvania State University College of Medicine (Hershey)
Perelman School of Medicine at the University of Pennsylvania (Philadelphia)
Temple University School of Medicine (Philadelphia)
The Commonwealth Medical College (Scranton)
University of Pittsburgh School of Medicine (Pittsburgh)

Puerto Rico
Ponce School of Medicine and Health Sciences (Ponce)
San Juan Bautista School of Medicine (Caguas)
Universidad Central del Caribe School of Medicine (Bayamon)
University of Puerto Rico School of Medicine (San Juan)

Rhode Island
The Warren Alpert Medical School of Brown University (Providence)

South Carolina
Medical University of South Carolina College of Medicine (Charleston)
University of South Carolina School of Medicine (Columbia)

South Dakota
Sanford School of Medicine The University of South Dakota (Sioux Falls)

Tennessee
East Tennessee State Univ. Quillen College of Medicine (Johnson City)
Meharry Medical College (Nashville)
University of Tennessee Health Science Center College of Medicine (Memphis)
Vanderbilt University School of Medicine (Nashville)

Texas
Baylor College of Medicine (Houston)
Texas A&M Health Science Center College of Medicine (Bryan)
Texas Tech Univ. Health Sciences Center Foster School of Medicine (El Paso)
Texas Tech Univ. Health Sciences Center School of Medicine (Lubbock)
The University of Texas School of Medicine at San Antonio (San Antonio)
University of Texas Medical Branch School of Medicine (Galveston)
University of Texas Medical School at Houston (Houston)
University of Texas Southwestern Medical Center (Dallas)

Utah
University of Utah School of Medicine (Salt Lake City)

Vermont
University of Vermont College of Medicine (Burlington)

Virginia
Eastern Virginia Medical School (Norfolk)
University of Virginia School of Medicine (Charlottesville)
Virginia Commonwealth University School of Medicine (Richmond)
Virginia Tech Carilion School of Medicine (Roanoke)

Washington
University of Washington School of Medicine (Seattle)

West Virginia
Marshall University Joan C. Edwards School of Medicine (Huntington)
West Virginia University School of Medicine (Morgantown)

Wisconsin
Medical College of Wisconsin (Milwaukee)
University of Wisconsin School of Medicine and Public Health (Madison)

Appendix C:
List of Osteopathic Medical Schools

Alabama
Alabama College of Osteopathic Medicine (Dothan)
Edward Via College of Osteopathic Medicine (Auburn)
Arkansas
Arkansas College of Osteopathic Medicine (Fort Smith)
Arizona
A.T. Still University–School of Osteopathic Medicine in Arizona (Mesa)
Arizona College of Osteopathic Medicine of Midwestern University
(Glendale)
California
Touro University College of Osteopathic Medicine–California (Vallejo)
Western University of Health Sciences/ College of Osteopathic Medicine of the
Pacific (Pomona)
Colorado
Rocky Vista University College of Osteopathic Medicine (Parker)
Florida
Lake Erie College of Osteopathic Medicine Bradenton Campus (Bradenton)
Nova Southeastern University College of Osteopathic Medicine (Fort
Lauderdale)
Georgia
Georgia Campus–Philadelphia College of Osteopathic Medicine (Suwanee)
Illinois
Chicago College of Osteopathic Medicine of Midwestern University (Downers
Grove)
Indiana
Marian University College of Osteopathic Medicine (Indianapolis)
Iowa
Des Moines University College of Osteopathic Medicine (Des Moines)
Kentucky
University of Pikeville Kentucky College of Osteopathic Medicine (Pikeville)
Maine
University of New England College of Osteopathic Medicine (Biddeford)
Michigan
Michigan State University College of Osteopathic Medicine (East Lansing)
Mississippi
William Carey University College of Osteopathic Medicine (Hattiesburg)
Missouri
A.T. Still University–Kirksville College of Osteopathic Medicine (Kirksville)
Kansas City University of Medicine and Biosciences College of Osteopathic
Medicine (Kansas City)

Nevada
Touro University Nevada College of Osteopathic Medicine (Henderson)
New Jersey
Rowan University School of Osteopathic Medicine (Stratford)
New Mexico
New Mexico State Univ. Burrell College of Osteopathic Medicine (Las Cruces)
New York
New York Institute of Technology College of Osteopathic Medicine (Old Westbury)
Touro College of Osteopathic Medicine–New York (New York City)
North Carolina
Campbell University School of Osteopathic Medicine (Buies Creek)
Ohio
Ohio University Heritage College of Osteopathic Medicine
(Athens)
Oklahoma
Oklahoma State University Center for Health Sciences College of Osteopathic Medicine (Tulsa)
Pennsylvania
Lake Erie College of Osteopathic Medicine (Erie)
Philadelphia College of Osteopathic Medicine (Philadelphia)
South Carolina
Edward Via College of Osteopathic Medicine–Carolinas Campus (Spartanburg)
Tennessee
Lincoln Memorial University–DeBusk College of Osteopathic Medicine (Harrogate)
Texas
University of Incarnate World School of Osteopathic Medicine (San Antonio)
University of North Texas Health Science Center at Fort Worth Texas College of Osteopathic Medicine (Ft. Worth)
Virginia
Edward Via College of Osteopathic Medicine–Virginia Campus (Blacksburg)
Liberty University College of Osteopathic Medicine (Lynchburg)
Washington
Pacific Northwest University of Health Sciences College of Osteopathic Medicine (Yakima)
West Virginia
West Virginia School of Osteopathic Medicine (Lewisburg)

www.ingramcontent.com/pod-product-compliance
Lightning Source LLC
Chambersburg PA
CBHW030918180526
45163CB00002B/390